Milady's Standard Nail Technology Exam Review

Catherine M. Frangie

Australia Canada Mexico Singapore Spain UnitedKingdom UnitedStates

Milady's Standard Nail Technology Exam Review
Catherine M. Frangie

Library of Congress Cataloging-in-Publication Data
ISBN-10: 1428359508
ISBN-13: 9781428359505

NOTICE TO THE READER

Publisher does not warrant or guarantee any of the products described herein or perform any independent analysis in connection with any of the product information contained herein. Publisher does not assume, and expressly disclaims, any obligation to obtain and include information other than that provided to it by the manufacturer.

The reader is expressly warned to consider and adopt all safety precautions that might be indicated by the activities herein and to avoid all potential hazards. By following the instructions contained herein, the reader willingly assumes all risks in connection with such instructions.

The Publisher makes no representation or warranties of any kind, including but not limited to, the warranties of fitness for particular purpose or merchantability, nor are any such representations implied with respect to the material set forth herein, and the publisher takes no responsibility with respect to such material. The publisher shall not be liable for any special, consequential, or exemplary damages resulting, in whole or part, from the readers' use of, or reliance upon, this material.

Milady's Standard
Nail Technology Exam Review

Foreword

This book of exam reviews contains questions similar to those that may be found on state licensing exams for nail technology. It employs the multiple-choice type question, which has been widely adopted and approved by the majority of state licensing boards.

Groups of questions have been arranged under major subject areas. To get the maximum advantage when using this book, it is advisable that the review of subject matter take place shortly after its classroom presentation.

This review book reflects advances in professional nail technology. It attempts to keep pace with, and insure a basic understanding of, sanitation, anatomy, physiology, and salon business applicable to the nail technician, client consultation guidelines, chemical safety in the nail salon, and basic manicuring and pedicuring procedures as well as some of the more advanced and creative aspects of the profession.

The book serves as an excellent guide for the student as well as for the experienced nail technician. It provides a reliable standard against which professionals can measure their knowledge, understanding, and abilities.

Furthermore, these reviews will help students and professionals alike to gain a more thorough understanding of the full scope of their work as they review practical performance skills and related theory. They will increase their ability to evaluate new products and procedures and to be better qualified professionals for dealing with the needs of their clients.

Part I: Exam Review for Nail Technology

CHAPTER 1—HISTORY AND OPPORTUNITIES

1. Define kosmetikos.
   a. skilled in the use of cosmetics
   b. cosmetologist
   c. esthetician
   d. nail technician
   _____

2. Which ancient civilization first created kohl makeup?
   a. Greeks
   b. Egyptians
   c. Chinese
   d. Romans
   _____

3. Different hair colors represented different classes in Roman society. Which of the following statements is NOT true?
   a. Blond indicated middle class.
   b. Black indicated lower class.
   c. Red was reserved for the nobility.
   d. Brown had a religious connotation
   _____

4. Queen Nefertiti _____ her nails with henna to create a rich red color.
   a. decorated
   b. polished
   c. stained
   d. airbrushed
   _____

5. If your calling is salon management, you can expect what type of responsibilities?
   a. inventory
   b. educator
   c. promotions
   d. all answers
   _____

6. Juliet wraps, a paper nail wrapping system, were applied with:
   a. nail resin
   b. acrylic
   c. gel
   d. airplane glue
   _____

7. Nail polish formulations have evolved to embody which of the following characteristics?
   a. chip-resistant
   b. fade-resistant
   c. lustrous finish
   d. all answers
   _____

8. What did Jeff Pink, founder of Orly International, create in 1975?
   a. French manicure
   b. Juliet wrap
   c. acrylic nails
   d. nail hardener
   _____

9. How do you achieve rapid success in the nail care business?
   a. focus on your studies
   b. attend workshops outside of school
   c. practice, practice, practice
   d. all answers
   _____

10. Charles Revson is so important to modern-day nail services because:
    a. he invented and marketed the first nail polish
    b. he invented nail polish
    c. he perfected top coat
    d. he was responsible for designing the first pair of nail nippers _____

11. In 1998, what groundbreaking system did Creative Nail Design introduce to the professional beauty market?
    a. the first spa pedicure system
    c. acrylic nail products
    b. nail tips
    d. the curette _____

12. We know that personal grooming and enhancement has been important since the dawn of history through archeological finds that include:
    a. mirrors, lip color, and combs
    b. animal sinew, sharpened flints, bones and oyster shells fashioned into combs and hair ornaments
    c. rawhide hair decorations
    d. tattoos for decoration _____

13. Among many firsts, the Egyptians were the first civilization to:
    a. cultivate beauty in an extravagant fashion
    c. use nail color
    b. extract essential oils
    d. paint their lips _____

14. The first known cosmetics factory was built by which famous beauty?
    a. Queen Cleopatra
    c. Gloria Swanson
    b. Queen Nefertiti
    d. Empress Eugenie _____

15. In 1600 B.C., a tinted mixture of gum arabic, gelatin, beeswax, and egg whites was used by Chinese aristocrats to:
    a. create eye makeup in dazzling colors
    b. color their nails crimson or ebony
    c. fortify their nails
    d. soften their skin _____

16. Egyptians used heavy amounts of kohl makeup to:
    a. alleviate eye inflammation
    c. beautify the eyes
    b. protect the eyes from glare
    d. all answers _____

17. Nail technicians have many career choices, including:
    a. distributor sales consultant
    c. retail sales and management
    b. editorial nail artist
    d. all answers _____

2

CHAPTER 2—LIFE SKILLS

1. The salon is a _____ by nature.
    a. customer-service oriented business
    b. place to exercise your creative talent
    c. highly social atmosphere
    d. all answers   _____

2. Game plan can best be defined as:
    a. the conscious act of planning your life
    b. always focusing on success
    c. knowing what you will be doing 1 month from now
    d. having goals that will further your career   _____

3. Staying on course for your entire career is much easier when you have_____.
    a. great life skills   c. consistency in your work
    b. good attitude   d. good concentration   _____

4. No matter how many hours you have worked, how should you greet your next client?
    a. by acting exhausted   c. with a handshake
    b. with the best smile   d. with genuine enthusiasm
        you can muster   _____

5. You should _____ any time studying for two hours at a stretch makes you feel overwhelmed.
    a. take a two-hour break   c. eat sugar and keep
             studying
    b. study in shorter chunks   d. condition yourself to study
        of time   for longer periods of time   _____

6. What stimulates clear thinking and career planning?
    a. competing in sports events   c. recreation and rest
    b. dancing and socializing   d. all answers   _____

7. Define "perfectionism."
    a. unhealthy desire to always be perfect
    b. ability to be perfect in certain things
    c. paying attention to detail
    d. appearing flawless   _____

8. Trusting in your ability to reach your goals is called:
    a. being conceited   c. an affirmation
    b. having good self-esteem   d. being self-absorbed   _____

9. Which of the following describe(s) sensitivity?
    a. understanding   c. acceptance
    b. empathy   d. all answers   _____

10. How should you prioritize your tasks when practicing time management?
    a. treat all tasks equally
    b. make a chart
    c. easiest to hardest
    d. most to least important _____

11. The most ideal place to study is:
    a. in a classroom where studying is the norm
    b. outdoors where the air is fresh and you can concentrate
    c. in a comfortable spot where you can lay down and feel relaxed
    d. in a quiet spot where you can study uninterrupted _____

12. Having _____can lead to a more satisfying and productive beauty career.
    a. a good education
    b. excellent social skills
    c. stamina
    d. great life skills _____

13. The salon is a highly social atmosphere requiring strong _____ in order to always act in a professional manner.
    a. sense of humor
    b. allies
    c. self-discipline
    d. family support _____

14. Listening attentively is:
    a. a trick
    b. tougher for men
    c. a natural talent
    d. a life skill _____

15. A necessary _____ is seeing jobs through to completion.
    a. life skill
    b. natural characteristic
    c. task
    d. talent _____

16. Guidelines for success can be defined as:
    a. principles that guide your behavior
    b. meditative phrases
    c. a set of beliefs
    d. guidelines for negative behavior _____

17. Respecting others is a:
    a. code of ethics
    b. guideline principle
    c. life skill
    d. rule of etiquette _____

18. Which of the following is NOT one of the 10 guiding principles?
    a. having all materials at the ready
    b. building self-esteem
    c. striving for excellence
    d. being consistent with your work _____

19. What is procrastination?
    a. not starting tasks until they are due
    b. putting off until tomorrow what you can do today
    c. being lazy
    d. delaying your success   ____

20. Every successful business follows what?
    a. a benefits manual   c. a monthly meeting plan
    b. a sound business plan   d. future plans   ____

21. What is the greatest benefit of setting goals?
    a. details your ambitions   c. helps determine your
                                       immediate needs
    b. keeps you organized   d. helps determine what you
                                       want out of life   ____

22. A long-term goal is which length of time?
    a. a week or longer   c. 5 years
    b. 6 months   d. 3 months   ____

23. Your mission statement should communicate:
    a. who you are; what you want out of life
    b. who you are; what you want others to think about you
    c. who you are; what you like
    d. who you are; how much money you want to earn   ____

24. Your personal mission statement should be read:
    a. every week   c. every day
    b. when you are stressed   d. three times a day   ____

25. Time management involves doing things in what order?
    a. least to most important   c. morning, afternoon, and
                                       evening activities
    b. most to least important   d. alphabetical order   ____

26. What does ethics mean?
    a. being faithful to your significant other
    b. moral principles that you live and work by
    c. never cheating on a test
    d. being a kind person   ____

27. Receptivity involves what?
    a. hearing clearly   c. being open-minded
    b. being a good listener   d. being empathetic   ____

28. What is diplomacy?
    a. being tactful   c. being aggressive
    b. being political   d. being assertive, but tactful ____

5

29. Good _____ means communicating clearly and directly with others.
    a. speaking skills   c. people skills
    b. communication skills   d. diction   _____

30. Define time management.
    a. saving enough time to study
    b. doing less things in more time
    c. making efficient use of your time
    d. doing more things in less time   _____

CHAPTER 3—YOUR PROFESSIONAL IMAGE

1. How you look and present yourself is important to your career because:
   a. you belong to the trend business
   b. it is part of looking professional
   c. you are in the image business
   d. dressing fashionably will build your clientele   ____

2. Define personal hygiene.
   a. daily maintenance of cleanliness through sanitary practices
   b. thorough hand washing
   c. wearing deodorant
   d. wearing clean, stain-free clothing   ____

3. What is a hygiene pack?
   a. pouch of hygiene products that should be kept at home
   b. pack you give to other stylists when they have bad breath or body odor
   c. pack that is only used during beauty school
   d. collection of personal hygiene products that you keep at your station or in your locker   ____

4. If you have bad body odor, what are clients most likely to do or say?
   a. hand you a breath mint
   b. say nothing, but continue to have you do their nails
   c. say nothing, but simply not return for another service
   d. tell you that you have offensive body odor and suggest that you do something about it   ____

5. Your hygiene pack should include a:
   a. toothbrush and toothpaste   c. hand sanitizer
   b. mouthwash   d. all answers   ____

6. What should you do if you smoke a cigarette before caring for a client?
   a. brush your teeth and use mouthwash
   b. wash hands
   c. use perfume
   d. brush your teeth, use mouthwash, and wash your hands   ____

7. Which of the following best applies to wearing perfume in the workplace?
   a. Keep perfume usage to a minimum, if at all.
   b. Wear only the latest fragrances.
   c. Only dab it behind your ears.
   d. Apply it only once a day.   ____

8. It is important for a nail technician to always have her hands and nails well manicured because it:
   a. lets others know you do fashion forward services
   b. inspires clients and instills confidence in your work
   c. helps you bond with the stylists
   d. increases the amount of tips per service   _____

9. In terms of hygiene, clothing should:
   a. be appropriate for your   c. look fresh and new
      figure
   b. be modest   d. be stain free and soil free   _____

10. _____ is an important part of having a good physical presentation.
    a. Good posture   c. Eloquent movements
    b. A pleasing walk   d. A graceful stride   _____

11. While doing nails, good posture includes:
    a. keeping legs and hips straight
    b. keeping head level with shoulders
    c. lifting upper body—do not slouch
    d. standing with your back straight   _____

12. Repetitive motion syndrome that results in injury to the wrist is called:
    a. carpal tunnel syndrome   c. phlebitis
    b. myofascial spasm   d. endocarpal syndrome   _____

13. Carpal tunnel syndrome can be partly avoided by:
    a. taking a 30-minute break between appointments
    b. using ergonomically designed implements
    c. gripping implements tightly
    d. keeping your elbows at least 60 degrees away from your body   _____

14. When performing nail services, always:
    a. bend forward to get closer to clients
    b. remember that clients' comfort comes first
    c. avoid bending forward; ask clients to move their hands or legs closer to you
    d. make sure that your chair supports your upper back   _____

15. What does ergonomics entail?
    a. sanitation practices
    b. OSHA regulations
    c. maximum comfort in the workplace
    d. designing the workplace for maximum comfort, safety, efficiency, and productivity of workers   _____

16. Which of the following has a cumulative effect on the muscles and joints:
    a. using an airbrush system
    b. rigid posture
    c. applying nail tips
    d. stressful, repetitive motions
    ____

17. What does dress code mean?
    a. maintaining an edgy appearance
    b. salon rules regarding the correct manner of dress for that particular business
    c. wearing only black or white
    d. wearing a uniform
    ____

18. Each year, hundreds of cosmetology professionals risk developing:
    a. inhibition of the circulatory system
    b. heart disease
    c. musculoskeletal disorders
    d. injury to the ulna
    ____

19. What is the guiding rule of makeup in the salon?
    a. maximize your best features
    b. only to be worn when you have time
    c. be edgy, even when the salon is not
    d. complement the colors of the salon
    ____

20. Define salon personality.
    a. personality of owner
    b. salon's overall image
    c. clients' preferences
    d. choice of music and decor
    ____

21. The best way to avoid developing a musculoskeletal disorder related to nail services is to:
    a. practice sound ergonomics
    b. never work more than 4 hours without a break
    c. do only three pedicures in an 8-hour day
    d. wear wrist guards while sleeping
    ____

22. Your clothing should always be clean, fresh, functional, and _____, whether or not you must abide by a salon dress code.
    a. cutting edge
    b. subdued
    c. embody the latest color trends
    d. stylish
    ____

23. When you work within the field of cosmetology, sitting improperly can put a great deal of _____ on your neck, shoulders, back and legs.
    a. weight
    b. muscles
    c. stress
    d. friction
    ____

24. The risk of developing repetitive motion syndrome of the wrist can be minimized by:
    a. using only titanium implements
    b. keeping your wrist vertical with the table
    c. keeping your wrist in a straight or neutral positon as much as possible
    d. using your right and left hands equally _____

25. To break up the repetitiveness of the motions you use, practice _____ to counter any physical discomfort.
    a. push-ups   c. pounding on a rubber mat
    b. juggling   d. regular stretching intervals _____

26. Which of the following is an example of ergonomic equipment?
    a. pedicure stool on rollers   c. manicure chair that can be raised and lowered
    b. halogen lamp   d. vibrating pedicure chair _____

27. You can convey an image of self-confidence when you:
    a. wear little to no makeup   c. give little thought to your appearance
    b. have good posture   d. wear a smock or apron _____

CHAPTER 4—COMMUNICATING FOR SUCCESS

1. You are in a better position to _____ when you clearly understand the motives and needs of others.
   a. make the right decisions
   b. do your job professionally and easily
   c. lend a sympathetic ear
   d. give good advice   _____

2. To build lasting client relationships and be a successful beauty professional, you must have great:
   a. personality traits
   b. communication skills
   c. mechanical skills
   d. chemistry   _____

3. The best way to _____ is to have a firm understanding of yourself.
   a. be attractive to the opposite sex
   b. be a great nail artist
   c. be certain of your career as a nail technician
   d. understand others   _____

4. What must you do to successfully handle difficult clients?
   a. Be aware of how you are feeling.
   b. Pay close attention to what clients are saying.
   c. Believe in yourself.
   d. All answers.   _____

5. When you and your client are both communicating clearly about an upcoming service:
   a. you are creating a fan club
   b. your chances of pleasing that client soar
   c. you will laugh more often
   d. you are showing patience with people   _____

6. The golden rules of human relations teach you to problem solve from your head and:
   a. communicate from your heart
   b. speak your mind
   c. avoid problems with your mind
   d. empathize with your soul   _____

7. When a tense situation arises, you should:
   a. react slowly
   b. avoid the situation
   c. act proactively
   d. remain calm   _____

8. When two people disagree on a certain subject, what should they do?
   a. debate until one concedes
   b. understand the other person's point of view
   c. stop talking
   d. be offended   _____

9. The golden rules of human relations stress the importance of knowing the difference between being right and being:
   a. wrong
   b. diplomatic
   c. narrow-minded
   d. righteous
   _____

10. What does communication mean?
    a. effectively sharing information
    b. talking clearly and loudly
    c. projecting your voice
    d. speaking the same language
    _____

11. Nail technicians communicate through words, voice inflections, facial expressions, body language, and:
    a. the quality of their own nails
    b. a sense of caring with clients
    c. visual tools
    d. finding common ground
    _____

12. A verbal communication that determines the desired results is called a:
    a. client consultation
    b. client intake form
    c. meet and greet
    d. client interview
    _____

13. A client consultation involves:
    a. learning about her lifestyle
    b. having an informal chat about her nails
    c. asking questions
    d. a structured fact-finding protocol
    _____

14. Repeating back what a client says using your own words is called:
    a. proactive listening
    b. reflective listening
    c. intuitive listening
    d. active listening
    _____

15. A quality client consultation does not include discussing a client's:
    a. lifestyle
    b. commitment
    c. personal problems
    d. personal style
    _____

16. How should you handle a tardy client when you still have time to do her nails?
    a. Let her know you can still do her nails because you happen to have a break in your schedule.
    b. Permanently remove her from your books.
    c. Teach her a lesson by not taking her.
    d. Take her and say nothing.
    _____

17. When dealing with an unhappy client, what should you never do?
    a. Give her choices to rectify the problem.
    b. If you cannot immediately fix the problem, tell her why.
    c. Argue with her.
    d. Empathize with her feelings. ____

18. Your job and your relationship with your clients are very specific; the goal is to advise and service clients with:
    a. emotional and professional support
    b. their beauty needs
    c. their problems
    d. personal advice ____

19. Which of the following answer(s) describe(s) professional salon behavior?
    a. being honest and sensitive
    b. treating everyone with respect
    c. keeping your private life private
    d. all answers ____

20. When you disagree with a salon policy, what should you do?
    a. Discuss this issue with your coworkers.
    b. Bring it up at a staff meeting.
    c. Respect and follow that rule.
    d. Circulate a petition. ____

21. An employee evaluation involves a:
    a. meeting where you are either fired or hired as a permanent employee
    b. performance evaluation
    c. checklist of salon faults
    d. checklist of your faults ____

22. A client intake form is a:
    a. financial form
    b. questionnaire that includes contact info, past history of nail services, and so on
    c. quiz about nail services
    d. list of clients' previous nail technicians and whether or not they were happy with their services ____

23. The manager's job in a salon situation is to:
    a. help with personal problems
    b. make sure the salon runs smoothly
    c. mediate conflicts between coworkers
    d. all answers ____

24. A(n) _____ cover health and lifestyle issues that could be contraindicative of having a nail service.
   a. consultation and intake form
   b. consultation and observing client's nails
   c. consultation and body language
   d. intake form and her body language   ____

25. During a nail consultation, which tool(s) should you be using?
   a. drawing of nail shapes   c. personal portfolio
   b. magazine clips   d. all answers   ____

CHAPTER 5—INFECTION CONTROL: PRINCIPLES AND PRACTICE

1. EPA stands for:
   a. Environmental Protection Agency
   b. Electric Power Agency
   c. Etiology and Pest Association
   d. Environment Protection Association   _____

2. What are the two primary types of bacteria?
   a. saprophytes and parasites
   b. pathogenic and nonpathogenic
   c. decomposing and fertilizing
   d. active and inactive   _____

3. _____ are plant or animal organisms that live in or on another living organism.
   a. Saprophytes
   b. Cocci
   c. Parasites
   d. Spore-forming bacteria   _____

4. When a disease spreads from one person to another by contact, it is said to be:
   a. contagious
   b. toxin
   c. inflamed
   d. spore-forming bacteria   _____

5. How many cells make up a bacterium?
   a. two cells
   b. one cell
   c. three molecules
   d. pathogenic   _____

6. _____ occurs when a bacterial cell divides into two new cells.
   a. Decomposing
   b. Fertilizing
   c. Mitosis
   d. Cell division   _____

7. A bacteria normally carried by about a third of the population is _____?
   a. staphylococci
   b. bacilli
   c. spirilla
   d. streptococci   _____

8. What type of microscopic organisms are capable of infecting almost all plants, animals, and bacteria?
   a. infections
   b. fungus
   c. parasites
   d. virus   _____

9. The pus-forming bacteria that grow in bunches or clusters are called:
   a. streptococci
   b. staphylococci
   c. bacilli
   d. pathogenic organisms   _____

10. An example of streptococci infection is:
    a. a boil
    c. a spherical spore
    b. a skin lesion
    d. blood poisoning
    _____

11. _____ gives us the ability to fight off or resist infections.
    a. Community resistance
    c. Immunity
    b. General infection
    d. Contagious infection
    _____

12. When you have immunity through inoculation or overcoming a disease, it is called:
    a. human disease resistor
    c. acquired immunity
    b. natural immunity
    d. acquired immune deficiency syndrome
    _____

13. Acquired immune deficiency syndrome or AIDS is caused by what virus?
    a. filterable bacteria
    c. HBV virus
    b. HIV
    d. filterable virus
    _____

14. Complete elimination of all microbial life, including spores, is called:
    a. sanitation
    c. removing bacteria
    b. sterilization
    d. laundering
    _____

15. Chemical agents that destroy all bacteria, fungi, and viruses, but not spores are called:
    a. disinfectants
    c. virucides
    b. styptic
    d. antiseptic
    _____

16. Identify the correct answer that lists all three steps of decontamination.
    a. sterilization, disinfection, sanitation
    b. disinfection, sanitation, laundering
    c. sterilization, disinfection, fumigation
    d. disinfection, sterilization, ultrasonic cleansing
    _____

17. You are _____ when you remove all visible dirt and debris from a surface.
    a. sterilizing
    c. sanitizing
    b. fumigating
    d. disinfecting
    _____

18. Putting antiseptics on your skin or washing your hands is another example of _____.
    a. sanitation
    c. sterilization
    b. disinfection
    d. immunity
    _____

19. _____ is the process that kills most, but not necessarily all, microoganisms on non-living surfaces.
    a. Fumigating   c. Sterilization
    b. Disinfection   d. Sanitizing   _____

20. HIV virus is spread mainly through:
    a. blood transfusions
    b. sharing hypodermic needles with intravenous drug users
    c. sexual contact with an infected person
    d. body fluids   _____

21. To properly disinfect your implements, they must be _____ for the prescribed amount of time.
    a. dipped   c. completely immersed
    b. washed   d. soaked   _____

22. The Hazard Communication Act does what?
    a. It requires chemical manufacturers and importers to assess the hazards associated with their products.
    b. Chemical manufacturers and importers no longer have to assess the hazards associated with their products.
    c. Licensed salon professionals must now assess the hazards associated with the products they are using.
    d. The salon owner is completely responsible for the hazards associated with any product they stock in their salon.   _____

23. Ethyl alcohol must be no less than a _____ strength to be an effective disinfectant.
    a. 70%   c. 80%
    b. 90%   d. 50%   _____

24. Sodium hypochlorite is the chemical name for this household staple:
    a. bathroom cleanser   c. phenolic disinfectant
    b. bleach   d. Lysol   _____

25. QUATS is short for what?
    a. quaternary antiseptic compounds
    b. quaternary ammonium compounds
    c. quaternary ammonium treatments
    d. quaternary antiseptic solutions   _____

26. Phenols may do what to certain rubber and plastic materials?
    a. damage   c. discolor and harden
    b. discolor and crack d. soften and tear   _____

27. What information do MSDS (Material Safety Data Sheets) provide about products?
    a. combustion levels   c. product content
    b. associated hazards   d. all answers   ____

28. The _____ approves all disinfectants in each state.
    a. OSHA   c. U.S. Department of Labor
    b. EPA   d. Chemists Society   ____

29. Bacteria thrive in _____ environments.
    a. warm, moist, dirty   c. cool, moist, dirty
    b. warm, dry, dirty   d. cool, dry, dirty   ____

30. In this stage, certain bacteria coat themselves with a wax outer shell in order to withstand unsuitable conditions.
    a. active   c. mitosis
    b. contagious   d. spore-forming   ____

31. What is a local infection?
    a. confined to a single area such as a pimple or abscess
    b. confined to one organ
    c. confined to the face, hands, or feet
    d. all answers   ____

32. What are bloodborne pathogens?
    a. disease-causing viruses   c. carried through the body in
                                     the blood or body fluids
    b. disease-causing bacteria   d. all answers   ____

33. What must a disinfectant be to meet salon disinfection standards?
    a. bactericidal, fungicidal, and virucidal
    b. pseudomonacidal, bactericidal, fungicidal, and pesticidal
    c. sterilizer, bactericidal, fungicidal, and virucidal
    d. disinfectant, bactericidal, fungicidal, and pesticidal   ____

34. Which answer(s) describe a phenolic disinfectant?
    a. corrosive material   c. caustic poison
    b. tuberculocidal disinfectant d. all answers   ____

35. A set of guidelines published by OSHA that require the employer and the employee to assume that all human blood and body fluids are infectious for bloodborne pathogens is called:
    a. Control of Infectious   c. Universal Precautions
       Diseases
    b. AIDs manual   d. Be Prepared Manual   ____

CHAPTER 6—GENERAL ANATOMY AND PHYSIOLOGY

1. Define anatomy.
   a. functions and activities performed by the body's structures
   b. minute structures of the body that cannot be seen with the naked eye
   c. structures of the body that can be seen with the naked eye
   d. the basic units of all living things _____

2. Identify the most important role that cells perform in the human body.
   a. constructive metabolism
   b. forming a protective covering on body surfaces
   c. mitosis
   d. carrying out all life processes _____

3. There are _____ of cells in the human body.
   a. millions
   b. trillions
   c. quadrillions
   d. quintillions _____

4. The composition of a cell does not include:
   a. protoplasm
   b. cytoplasm
   c. catabolism
   d. nucleus _____

5. Cell metabolism is composed of two phases:
   a. anabolism and canabolism
   b. anabolism and catabolism
   c. cathartic and lethargic
   d. libation and privation _____

6. How many types of tissues are found in the human body?
   a. five
   b. ten
   c. hundreds
   d. three _____

7. The connective tissue's primary role is to:
   a. support, protect, and bind together other tissues of the body
   b. support, protect, and bind together different types of keratin
   c. protect against aging skin
   d. aid in coordination _____

8. Identify the primary role(s) of nerve tissues:
   a. carry messages to and from the brain; control all body functions
   b. carry messages to and from the organs; control organ functions
   c. carry messages to and from the heart, kidneys, and lungs
   d. keep the heart beating _____

9. Identify the role(s) of muscle tissue in the human body:
    a. balances the body; allows you to move
    b. allows you to make skilled movements; allows you to sit upright
    c. contracts and moves various parts of the body
    d. causes eye tics   _____

10. The _____ excrete(s) water and waste products.
    a. liver   c. stomach
    b. pancreas   d. kidneys   _____

11. Which is not a system of the body?
    a. circulatory   c. endocrine
    b. pancreatic   d. all answers   _____

12. What is the skeletal system?
    a. gives form to the human body
    b. made up of bones and movable and immovable joints
    c. protects internal organs
    d. serves as attachments for muscles   _____

13. How many bones are there in the human skeletal system?
    a. 206   c. 226
    b. 260   d. 602   _____

14. Identify three movable joints.
    a. elbows, knees, and hips   c. ulna, radius, and carpus
    b. pelvis, wrists, and ankles   d. elbows, knees, and fingers   _____

15. Define osteology.
    a. bone disease   c. study of bones
    b. study of ligaments   d. study of the hardness of
                                           bones   _____

16. Muscles are made of what?
    a. millions of tiny protein   c. millions of epithelial cells
        filaments
    b. millions of ligaments   d. tough, fibrous tissue   _____

17. What is the humerus?
    a. uppermost, largest bone of the arm
    b. inner bone of the forearm
    c. smaller bone on the thumb side of forearm
    d. largest palm bone   _____

18. Define myology.
    a. study of the nature, structure, and function of the bones
    b. study of the nature, structure, function, and diseases of the nerves
    c. study of the structure, function, and diseases of the muscles
    d. study of the nature, structure, and function of the human body   _____

19. The study of the nervous system and its disorders is called:
    a. histology   c. osteology
    b. neurology   d. trichology   _____

20. The three main subdivisions of the nervous system are:
    a. central, peripheral, and autonomic
    b. central, peripheral, and metabolic
    c. spinal, peripheral, and automatic
    d. central, sensory, and motor   _____

21. Which part of the cell body receives messages from other neurons?
    a. axon   c. axon terminal
    b. dendrite   d. nucleus   _____

22. The nervous system's primary structural units are called:
    a. mixed nerves   c. neurons
    b. afferents   d. efferents   _____

23. The sensory and motor nerve fibers that carry impulses or messages to and from the central nervous system to all parts of the body make up the:
    a. peripheral nervous system c. parasympathetic system
    b. autonomic nervous system   d. central nervous system   _____

24. What is the role of the adductors?
    a. draw the fingers together   c. protect against rheumatoid arthritis
    b. spread the fingers   d. move the fingers from side to side   _____

25. The little finger side of the arm and the palm of the hand are supplied by the _____ nerve and its branches.
    a. digital   c. median
    b. radial   d. ulnar   _____

26. Which parts of the heart are responsible for allowing the blood to flow in only one direction?
    a. atria   c. valves
    b. ventricles   d. arteries   _____

27. The sticky, salty fluid that circulates throughout the circulatory system is called:
    a. white corpuscles
    b. blood
    c. plasma
    d. red corpuscles
    _____

28. What do red and white blood cells and blood platelets flow through?
    a. white corpuscles
    b. plasma
    c. red corpuscles
    d. lymph
    _____

29. What percentage of water is found in plasma?
    a. 60 percent
    b. 70 percent
    c. 80 percent
    d. 90 percent
    _____

30. What is the process of breaking down food into nutrients that can be used by the body?
    a. exhalation
    b. digestion
    c. evacuation
    d. contraction
    _____

31. Which organ is responsible for converting certain elements from the blood into new compounds?
    a. endocrines
    b. glands
    c. exocrines
    d. carotids
    _____

32. The _____ system is another name for the digestive system.
    a. excretory
    b. elimination
    c. integumentary
    d. gastrointestinal
    _____

33. What separates the chest from the abdominal region and controls breathing?
    a. pericardium
    b. chest cavity
    c. rib cage
    d. diaphragm
    _____

34. The basic unit of all living things is called a:
    a. nucleus
    b. cell
    c. protoplasm
    d. neuron
    _____

35. For cells to reproduce, what must be in place?
    a. the right temperature
    b. the ability to eliminate
    c. adequate supplies of food, oxygen, and water
    d. all answers
    _____

36. The role of cell metabolism is to:
    a. produce more daughter cells
    b. provide cell nourishment
    c. enable cells to reproduce
    d. keep the cells from turning into fat cells
    _____

37. What does catabolism do?
    a. breaks down fat cells
    b. breaks down proteins so that they can be absorbed by other cells
    c. breaks down complex compounds within cells into smaller ones
    d. builds large molecules from smaller ones   _____

38. How do cells react to unfavorable conditions such as toxins and disease?
    a. cells become bloated
    b. they do not affect cells
    c. metabolism is increased within the cell
    d. cells become impaired or die   _____

39. What is mitosis?
    a. human reproduction
    b. glandular reproduction
    c. cell reproduction
    d. saliva reproduction   _____

40. Fascia, ligaments, fat, and tendons are _____ tissue.
    a. connective
    b. protective
    c. integumentary
    d. muscular   _____

41. What components are found in liquid tissue?
    a. lymph and white corpuscles
    b. blood and lymph
    c. saliva and blood
    d. red corpuscles and bile   _____

42. Lungs supply the blood with:
    a. hydrogen
    b. nitrous oxide
    c. carbon dioxide
    d. oxygen   _____

43. What is the role of the digestive system?
    a. breaks down gases
    b. changes food into nutrients and wastes
    c. sorts out different kinds of waste
    d. keeps your system well fed   _____

44. The heart and blood vessels comprise which system?
    a. blood system
    b. not part of a system
    c. respiratory system
    d. circulatory system   _____

45. The muscular system:
    a. allows the body to move
    b. contracts and moves various parts of the body
    c. allows for skilled movements
    d. makes motor function possible   _____

46. The body's hardest substance can be found in the:
    a. bones
    b. skull
    c. teeth
    d. pelvis
    _____

47. The human body has _____ muscles.
    a. over 1,000
    b. over 300
    c. over 600
    d. about 100
    _____

48. All these pertain to the makeup of muscles except:
    a. origin
    b. epithelial
    c. belly
    d. insertion
    _____

49. What are striated muscles?
    a. attached to the bone and are voluntarily controlled
    b. involuntary heart muscles
    c. involuntary muscles found in internal organs
    d. all answers
    _____

50. The hand's two most important muscles are:
    a. abductors and adductors
    b. pronators and supinators
    c. pectoralis major and pectoralis minor
    d. flexors and extensors
    _____

51. Muscles are fibrous tissue that have the ability to:
    a. stretch but not contract
    b. contract but not stretch
    c. stretch and contract
    d. none of the choices available
    _____

52. What are the functions of the latissimus dorsi?
    a. control the shoulder blade and swinging movements of the arm
    b. control the neck and swinging movements of the arm
    c. control the hips and swinging movements of the legs
    d. control the trapezius muscle and swinging movements of the arms
    _____

53. The _____ assists in breathing and raising the arm.
    a. diaphragm
    b. deltoid
    c. serratus anterior
    d. triceps
    _____

54. The sensory nerves:
    a. carry impulses from sense organs to the brain
    b. enable you to sense touch, cold, and heat
    c. enable you to experience sight, hearing, taste, smell, and pain
    d. all answers
    _____

24

55. What is the most important function of the lymph vascular system?
    a. aids in digestion
    b. carries waste and impurities away from the cells
    c. nourishes the cells
    d. protects against Hodgkin's disease
    _____

56. Which nerve and its branches supply the fingers?
    a. digital nerve   c. ulnar nerve
    b. radial nerve   d. median nerve
    _____

57. The pulmonary system and the _____ are responsible for carrying blood throughout the body.
    a. recirculating system   c. lymph system
    b. systemic or general   d. hemoglobin
       circulation system
    _____

58. What are the names of the two main arteries that supply blood to the hand?
    a. major and minor   c. red and blue
    b. ulnar and radial   d. pulmonary and circulatory
                                 system
    _____

59. The platelets:
    a. aid in digestion   c. prevent anemia
    b. aid in blood clotting d. fight infections
    _____

60. The _____ defends against invading microorganisms and toxins.
    a. red corpuscle   c. liver
    b. lymph vascular system d. pancreas
    _____

CHAPTER 7—SKIN STRUCTURE AND GROWTH

1. Which of the following is the largest organ of the body?
   a. intestines
   b. hair
   c. integumentary system
   d. skin _____

2. The _____ consists of the stratum spinosum, stratum lucidum, and stratum corneum.
   a. epidermis
   b. subcutaneous
   c. dermis
   d. hypodermis _____

3. Blood vessels, nerves, sweat glands, and oil glands are found in which layer of the skin?
   a. dermis
   b. epidermis
   c. subdermis
   d. stratum corneum _____

4. How is skin nourished?
   a. Oxygen and nutrients are carried through the bloodstream.
   b. Proteins and fats are carried through the lymphatic system.
   c. Enzymes provide skin with nourishment.
   d. Skin does not need nourishment. _____

5. The dermis is also called:
   a. true skin
   b. cutis
   c. corium
   d. all answers _____

6. The _____ has nerve endings but no blood vessels.
   a. dermis
   b. hypodermis
   c. epidermis
   d. papillary _____

7. What is the primary purpose of the subcutaneous tissue?
   a. contains fats for use as energy
   b. acts as a protective cushion
   c. gives smoothness and contour to the body
   d. all answers _____

8. The two types of pigment found in the skin are:
   a. pheomelanin and eumelanin
   b. red and yellow melanin
   c. brown and black melanin
   d. island of melanin, lentigo _____

9. Nerve endings are most abundant in the:
   a. knuckles
   b. fingertips
   c. palm
   d. dorsal _____

10. What are collagen and elastin?
    a. flexible ligaments that hold the skin together.
    b. flexible protein fibers found within the dermis.
    c. fibrous bands that anchor the skin to the subcutaneous layer
    d. cells that help protect the skin against UV rays ____

11. Define the function of collagen:
    a. helps skin regain its shape
    b. provides form and strength to the skin
    c. is more abundant in adults
    d. eliminates redness in the skin ____

12. Which of the following are lifestyle habits that cause premature aging of the skin?
    a. excessive alcohol consumption
    b. smoking
    c. overexposure to UV rays
    d. all answers ____

13. _____ duct glands extract materials from the blood to form new substances.
    a. Sudoriferous and sebaceous
    b. Sudoriferous and arrector pili
    c. Liver and pancreas
    d. Sudoriferous and lymph ____

14. The glands that eliminate up to two pints of liquid daily are called:
    a. sebaceous glands
    b. sudoriferous glands
    c. livers
    d. skin ____

15. Body temperature is regulated by this gland:
    a. circulatory
    b. integumentary
    c. sudoriferous
    d. endocrine ____

16. The #1 cause of skin aging is long-term exposure to:
    a. sun
    b. fluorescent lights
    c. makeup
    d. gravity ____

17. It is very important that a salon does not serve a client who is suffering from:
    a. moles that have changed color, size, or shape
    b. pigmented spots that have irregular borders
    c. skin that unexpectedly bleeds or will not heal quickly
    d. all answers ____

18. After swimming or water play, what should you do?
    a. nothing if you are wearing a broad-spectrum sunscreen
    b. apply just a little sunscreen
    c. avoid applying sunscreen unless your sunscreen is not water resistant.
    d. reapply recommended amount of sunscreen ____

19. Which of the following professionals is qualified to diagnose a skin disorder?
    a. esthetician   c. physician
    b. nurse practitioner   d. pharmacist ____

20. A bulla is a(n):
    a. large blister containing   c. inflamed, pus-filled pimple
       watery fluid
    b. round solid lump   d. flat, discolored spot ____

21. A wheal is a(n):
    a. abnormal mass caused by excessive multiplication of cells
    b. closed, fluid-filled mass below the surface of the skin
    c. itchy, swollen lesion that lasts a few hours
    d. small blister or sac containing clear fluid ____

22. What are flaky, dry, or oily scales such as dandruff called?
    a. ulcers   c. fissures
    b. scales   d. cicatrix ____

23. Define excoriation.
    a. deep lesion   c. gash
    b. superficial scratch d. rash ____

24. Define comedo.
    a. whitehead   c. hair follicle filled with
                       keratin and sebum
    b. blackhead   d. milia ____

25. Dilated capillaries called _____ can be caused by tobacco use, sun exposure, or other environmental factors.
    a. halitosis   c. rosacea
    b. seborrheic dermatitis   d. telangiectasias ____

26. Miliaria rubra is the medical name for:
    a. inability to sweat   c. prickly heat
    b. offensive body odor   d. psoriasis ____

27. Dermatitis is a(n):
   a. contagious skin rash
   b. inflammation of the skin caused by an allergic reaction or skin irritant
   c. condition characterized by silver-white scales
   d. form of eczema _____

28. Which type of dermatitis is the most common skin disease for nail technicians?
   a. formaldehyde dermatitis
   c. general dermatitis
   b. mite-related dermatitis
   d. contact dermatitis _____

29. How can clients develop contact dermatitis to a nail ingredient?
   a. being exposed to fumes during acrylic nail services
   b. being exposed to a sensitizing nail product over a long period of time
   c. systemic reaction unrelated to exposure
   d. nail ingredients are natural sensitizers _____

30. Nail technicians are most likely to develop contact dermatitis in which area(s)?
   a. between thumb and index finger
   c. back of forearm
   b. palms
   d. all answers _____

31. Clients can eventually develop contact dermatitis to nail products when nail technicians:
   a. do not leave a 1/16" free margin between the product and skin
   b. apply a dry product ratio-mix to the nail
   c. apply an overly thin coat of gel product
   d. overcure their UV gel nail enhancements _____

32. _____ is the most common type and least severe form of skin cancer.
   a. Malignant melanoma
   c. Basal cell carcinoma
   b. Squamous cell carcinoma
   d. Skin tags _____

33. To ensure that your UV bulbs are adequately curing gel nail enhancements, you should:
   a. replace bulbs at least three times per year
   b. clean surfaces of bulbs on a daily basis
   c. use the lamp designed for your system
   d. all answers _____

34. A mark on the skin indicating an injury or damage that caused a structural change in tissue is called a:
   a. bulla
   b. macule
   c. lesion
   d. papule
   _____

35. What do bleach, strong cleaning agents, quats, solvents, and acetone have in common?
   a. too caustic for salon use
   b. potential skin irritants
   c. sanitizing agents
   d. diluted products
   _____

36. Nail technicians can avoid developing contact dermatitis by:
   a. wiping their table down after each client
   b. practicing meticulous sanitary practices
   c. wearing gloves when using acetone to remove nail polish
   d. wiping down products on a daily basis
   _____

37. What is a keratoma?
   a. bruise
   b. welt
   c. type of skin cancer
   d. callus
   _____

38. What does vitiligo look like?
   a. multihued warts
   b. blackening of the skin
   c. dark and light spots
   d. milky-white spots
   _____

39. What is the role of an antioxidant?
   a. can prevent certain types of cancer
   c. aids free radicals
   b. works against natural skin function
   d. contributes to DNA damage within skin cells
   _____

40. A medical term for abnormal skin inflammation is called:
   a. overexposure
   b. dermatitis
   c. sensitization
   d. histamines
   _____

41. Healthy skin should contain between _____ of water.
   a. 85 and 90 percent
   b. 45 and 55 percent
   c. 50 and 70 percent
   d. 75 and 77 percent
   _____

42. When cells become dehydrated, what happens to them?
   a. Skin becomes weathered looking.
   b. They become stronger.
   c. They make more collagen.
   d. They cannot function properly.
   _____

43. Even mild dehydration can cause:
   a. rapid aging
   b. daytime fatigue
   c. memory loss
   d. all answers
   _____

44. You can lessen hunger without consuming calories by:
    a. putting it out of your mind   c. drinking a glass of water
    b. smelling the food you crave   d. speeding up your
                                          metabolism
                                                                    _____

CHAPTER 8—NAIL STRUCTURE AND GROWTH

1. Nails are appendages of the skin and therefore part of the
    _____ system.
    a. skeletal
    b. integumentary
    c. endocrine
    d. muscular ____

2. A dehydrated nail:
    a. is weak
    b. is brittle
    c. has a yellow tinge
    d. cannot grow past the free
        edge ____

3. How can you improve the water content of dehydrated nails?
    a. Have clients drink 8 glasses of water a day.
    b. Have clients use hand cream every night.
    c. Use a cuticle cream every morning.
    d. Treat the nail plate with an oil-based nail conditioner and
        keep the nails polished. ____

4. The natural nail is composed mainly of _____.
    a. melanin
    b. keratin
    c. several different proteins
    d. calcium ____

5. A healthy nail should contain _____ water.
    a. 14 percent
    b. 10 percent
    c. 30 to 50 percent
    d. 15 to 25 percent ____

6. A thin layer tissue called the bed epithelium _____
    and helps guide the nail as it grows.
    a. creates deep folds of skin around nail plate
    b. anchors the nail plate to the nail bed
    c. anchors nail bed to the underlying bone
    d. provides the underlying support for the nail plate ____

7. The visible part of the matrix that extends from underneath the
    living skin is called the:
    a. cuticle
    b. eponychium
    c. lunula
    d. hyponychium ____

8. What forms the nail plate?
    a. hyponychium
    b. epithelial tissue
    c. keratin
    d. matrix cells ____

9. Poor nail growth can be caused by what?
    a. poor general health
    b. injury to the matrix
    c. nail disorder or disease
    d. all answers ____

10. The nail plate consists of approximately _____ layers.
    a. 10   c. 500
    b. 100   d. 1,000   _____

11. The matrix is vital to the nail plate because:
    a. it prevents fungus from infesting the nail bed
    b. it is where the natural nail is formed
    c. it is the most active part of the skin
    d. nail growth would be sluggish without it   _____

12. The primary purpose of the cuticle is to:
    a. do nothing   c. hold the nail in place
    b. help shape the nail   d. protect against injury and
                                infection   _____

13. The fastest nail growth is experienced by:
    a. men   c. children
    b. women   d. young adults   _____

14. Which season is credited for fastest nail growth?
    a. summer   c. winter
    b. spring   d. fall   _____

15. What influences the thickness, width, and curvature of the
    nail?
    a. length, width, and curvature of the matrix
    b. length, width, and curvature of the nail bed
    c. length, width, and curvature of the nail folds
    d. thickness, width, and curvature of the matrix   _____

16. The _____ nail grows the fastest.
    a. middle finger   c. index
    b. thumb   d. all nails grow the same   _____

17. A tough band of fibrous tissue that attach the nail bed and the
    matrix bed to underlying bone is called:
    a. cuticle   c. eponychium
    b. hyponychium   d. specialized ligaments   _____

18. It takes approximately _____ for the nail to grow from the
    base to the free edge.
    a. 4 to 6 months   c. 9 months
    b. 1 month   d. 1 year   _____

19. How long does it take for a toenail to grow from the base of
    the nail bed to the free edge?
    a. 3 to 4 years   c. 9 months to a year
    b. 3 to 6 months   d. 6 months to a year   _____

20. A highly curved nail is caused by what?
    a. flat nail bed   c. highly curved free edge
    b. injury   d. highly curved matrix   _____

21. The average adult fingernail grows _____ in 1 month.
    a. 1/10 inch   c. 1/8 inch
    b. 1/4 inch   d. 1/3 inch   _____

22. Nail growth is affected by:
    a. nutrition   c. general health
    b. exercise   d. all answers   _____

23. How does an adequate water content affect nails?
    a. toughens nails   c. makes nails less flexible
    b. makes nails more flexible d. allows polish to remain
       true to color   _____

24. What is the purpose of nail grooves or tracks?
    a. Nails move along these   c. They do not exist.
       tracks as they grow.
    b. They signal poor health.   d. They anchor the nail. _____

CHAPTER 9—NAIL DISEASES AND DISORDERS

1. When living skin splits around the nail, it is called:
   a. melanonychia
   b. hangnail
   c. furrow
   d. beau's break
   ____

2. A trumpet or pincer nail is a(n):
   a. scarring of the distal nail fold
   b. horizontal nail depression
   c. extremely thin and weak nail
   d. highly exaggerated nail curvature
   ____

3. What does nail psoriasis do to the nails?
   a. pits the nails
   b. causes onychorrhexis
   c. causes onychocryptosis
   d. causes onychophagy
   ____

4. Leukonychia spots are:
   a. a potentially fatal form of cancer
   b. a direct result of contact dermatitis
   c. white spots not related to health
   d. caused by calcium deficiency
   ____

5. Describe a bruised nail.
   a. White spots appear on nail plate.
   b. Purplish blood clot forms under the nail.
   c. Nail bed goes from blue to green.
   d. Nail has a bruised appearance for three days or less.
   ____

6. Discolored nails turn a variety of colors and may indicate a/an:
   a. systemic disorder, poor blood circulation
   b. too much beta carotene
   c. injury to the matrix
   d. poor lifestyle choices
   ____

7. Define onychocryptosis.
   a. a plicatured nail
   b. dark ridges
   c. infected ingrown nail
   d. ingrown nail
   ____

8. The pressure of an ingrown nail can be relieved by doing what?
   a. filing the nail corners square
   b. cutting away the sides of the nail
   c. gently curving the corners of the nail
   d. cutting the nail very short
   ____

9. When filing eggshell nails, what grit should you use?
   a. 240 grit or higher
   b. 80 grit
   c. 100 grit
   d. should not file at all
   ____

10. A nail disease more susceptible to bartenders, health care workers and food processors.
    a. onychia
    b. nail psoriasis
    c. onycholysis
    d. paronychia

    ____

11. What is another term for onychophagy?
    a. incurable fungus
    b. bitten nails
    c. onychocryptosis
    d. melanoma

    ____

12. Which of the following cause(s) beau's lines?
    a. pneumonia
    b. adverse drug reaction
    c. heart failure
    d. all answers

    ____

13. What is onychia?
    a. green spot between the natural nail and the nail enhancement
    b. eggshell nails
    c. inflammation around the matrix
    d. abnormal damage to the eponychium

    ____

14. What causes onychia?
    a. improperly disinfected nail implements
    b. waiting too long between nail appointments
    c. nail polish remover
    d. double-dipping a nail brush during a nail service

    ____

15. Define fungi.
    a. Parasites that cause bad foot odor.
    b. Parasites that can infect the hands and feet.
    c. Green parasites.
    d. Parasites that lead to bacterial infections.

    ____

16. The discoloration that sometimes develops between the nail plate and the nail enhancement is caused by:
    a. mold
    b. fungus
    c. bacteria
    d. dirt

    ____

17. An advanced bacterial infection between the nail plate and an artificial nail enhancement is _____ in color.
    a. yellow-green
    b. brown
    c. orange
    d. brown-black

    ____

18. How should you treat a client's fungus infection?
    a. Scrub the nail, soak in quats.
    b. Spray with a fungicide solution.
    c. Apply an antifungal cream.
    d. Refer to a physician.

    ____

19. Define onychomycosis.
    a. mold infection of the natural nail plate
    b. bacterial infection of the natural nail plate
    c. fungal infection of the natural nail plate
    d. none of the choices listed _____

20. _____ is the separation and falling off of a nail plate from the nail bed.
    a. Nail psoriasis   c. Paronychia
    b. Onychia   d. Onychomadesis _____

21. What is the medical name for a foot fungus?
    a. tinea digitata   c. tinea pedis
    b. pedius fungi   d. tinea digiti _____

22. Ridges running vertically down the length of the natural nail plate are caused by:
    a. leukemia   c. overheating
    b. age   d. dehydration _____

23. Paronychia is more prevalent on the:
    a. toenails   c. big toes
    b. fingernails   d. thumbs _____

24. How should you treat nails that are brittle, are deeply split, and have vertical ridges?
    a. Fill split with fast-drying glue.
    b. Treat only if nail is not split down to the nail bed.
    c. Apply ridge filler.
    d. Buff away ridges, avoiding the split area. _____

25. A fungal infection called tinea pedis can be described as:
    a. itchy red rash between   c. small blisters
       the toes
    b. flaking   d. all answers _____

26. Define pyogenic granuloma.
    a. a serious condition that contributes to several types of cancer, especially melanoma
    b. severe infection characterized by a lump of red tissue growing up from the nail bed to the nail plate
    c. mild infection characterized by a lump of pink tissue growing up from the nail bed to the nail plate
    d. a parasitic condition that begins as a mild fungal infection, and grows worse over time _____

27. What are the attributes of a healthy nail?
    a. firm, inflexible, shiny, and slightly pink or yellow.
    b. flexible, shiny, thick, and slightly pink or yellow
    c. firm, flexible, shiny, and slightly pink or yellow
    d. firm, inflexible, thick, and slightly pink or yellow
    ____

28. A _____ is a condition caused by injury or disease.
    a. healthy nail   c. fungus
    b. mold   d. nail disorder
    ____

29. As a professional it is important to carefully study nail
    structure, nail diseases and disorders for:
    a. your safety
    b. your client's safety
    c. your safety, your client's safety, and the safety of those
       around you
    d. safety of those around you
    ____

30. This bacterial infection is incorrectly referred to as mold.
    a. Pseudomonas aerobica   c. Pseudomonas botanica
    b. Pseudomonas aeruginosa   d. Pseudomonas prolifica
    ____

31. While services are being performed, fungi and bacteria can be
    spread by:
    a. sneezing   c. unsanitary implements
    b. improper sanitation and   d. not using antibacterial
       disinfection practices   soap when washing hands   ____

32. You should decline to do a nail service any time:
    a. there is inflamed or infected skin
    b. there is broken skin or swelling
    c. a condition is present that may be contagious
    d. all answers
    ____

33. It is safe to perform nail services when this condition is
    present:
    a. onychosis   c. onychia
    b. onychophagy   d. paronychia
    ____

34. Cutting off living tissue during a manicure causes _____
    to develop.
    a. hangnails   c. eggshell nails
    b. furrows   d. white spots
    ____

35. Abnormal condition that occurs when skin is stretched by the
    nail plate.
    a. scalp ringworm   c. honeycomb ringworm
    b. athlete's foot   d. nail pterygium
    ____

36. Onycholysis is caused by:
    a. physical injury
    b. allergic reaction of the nail bed
    c. health disorder
    d. all answers

    ____

37. What does onycholysis cause the nail to do?
    a. break off at the free edge
    b. fall off
    c. lift away from the nail bed without shedding
    d. discolor and crumble

    ____

CHAPTER 10—BASICS OF CHEMISTRY

1. Solid matter:
   a. has volume but not shape
   b. has shape and form
   c. lacks shape and volume
   d. has only volume ____

2. Matter exists in which forms?
   a. minerals and water
   b. solid, liquid, and gas
   c. water and oxygen
   d. nitrous oxide and gas ____

3. All matter is composed of:
   a. atoms
   b. carbon
   c. compounds
   d. hydrogen ____

4. Define element.
   a. solid
   b. simplest form of matter
   c. compound
   d. unique molecules ____

5. Define organic chemistry.
   a. study of nonchemical substances
   b. study of substances containing vegetable matter
   c. study of pesticide-free foods
   d. study of substances containing carbon ____

6. Which of the following best describes carbon?
   a. metallic element found in all living things
   b. a substance found in all living things, or things that were once alive, whether plant or animal
   c. naturally occurring element
   d. a form of energy ____

7. Define inorganic substances.
   a. substances like gas, oil, and coal
   b. substances that have never been alive
   c. all minerals
   d. water, air, and metals ____

8. How many naturally occurring elements are there in the universe?
   a. 112
   b. 93
   c. 100
   d. 90 ____

9. Define atom.
   a. particles from which all matter is composed
   b. particles from which most matter is composed
   c. particles from which natural matter is composed
   d. particles from which inorganic matter is composed ____

10. Define physical property.
    a. color, odor, weight, and density
    b. characteristics determined without a chemical reaction
    c. chemical change
    d. changing form without forming a new substance   _____

11. What are elemental molecules?
    a. two or more atoms of the same element that have been
       united physically
    b. aluminum foil
    c. two or more atoms of different elements that are united
       chemically
    d. substances made up of elements that have been combined
       physically, rather than chemically (e.g., concrete).   _____

12. Identify one or more physical mixtures.
    a. concrete   c. cornbread
    b. saltwater   d. all answers   _____

13. A physical mixture that contains two or more different
    substances is called:
    a. a solution   c. an emulsion
    b. a suspension   d. all answers   _____

14. Define solute.
    a. certain miscible liquids   c. solvent
    b. a substance that is   d. solution
       dissolved in a solution   _____

15. What is a suspension?
    a. solid particles distributed throughout a liquid medium that
       tend to separate over time
    b. surfactant
    c. moisture of two or more immiscible substances united with
       the aid of a binder or emulsifier
    d. immiscible liquid   _____

16. Define solution.
    a. solute
    b. a stable mixture of two or more mixable substances
    c. two pure substances blended together
    d. surfactant   _____

17. Describe the head of a surfactant.
    a. hydrophilic or water loving and dissolves in water
    b. lipophilic or oil loving and dissolves in oil
    c. neither water loving nor oil loving
    d. dissolves in both water and oil to form an emulsion   _____

18. Water-in-oil emulsions are:
    a. ointments
    b. oil droplets that are suspended in a water base
    c. surfactants
    d. water droplets that are suspended in an oil base   ____

19. Oil-in-water emulsions have:
    a. a much greater amount of oil
    b. a much greater amount of water
    c. slightly more water than oil
    d. slightly more oil than water   ____

20. Which of the following would be considered a pure substance?
    a. atoms   c. elements
    b. compound molecules   d. all answers   ____

21. What is the purpose of glycerin?
    a. used as a solvent and a moisturizer in body creams
    b. used to neutralize acids
    c. used in place of ammonia to raise the pH
    d. used as a water-resistant lubricant   ____

22. Substances that act as a bridge to allow oil and water to mix, or emulsify.
    a. element   c. redox
    b. emulsion   d. surfactants   ____

23. Which of the following is the most complete definition of an ion?
    a. an atom or molecule that carries a negative electrical charge
    b. an atom or molecule that carries an electrical charge
    c. an ion with a positive electrical charge
    d. a cation under certain circumstances   ____

24. Water molecules naturally ionize into _____ and _____.
    a. Hydrogen ions and anion ions.
    b. Water molecules do not ionize.
    c. Hydrogen ions and hydroxide ions.
    d. Hydrogen ions and cation ions.   ____

25. Which ions are measured by the pH scale?
    a. water molecules that have naturally ionized into hydrogen ions and some into hydroxide ions
    b. only water molecules that have ionized into hydroxide ions
    c. water molecules that have ionized into cation and anion ions
    d. only water molecules that have ionized into hydrogen ions   ____

26. What does the pH scale measure?
    a. the acidity of a liquid
    b. the alkalinity of a liquid
    c. both the acidic and alkaline quality of a substance
    d. the degree of acidity or alkalinity of aqueous solutions   ____

27. The pH scale ranges from:
    a. 0 to 15   c. 0 to 12
    b. 0 to 14   d. 0 to 10   ____

28. What does 7 represent on the pH scale?
    a. acidic pH   c. alkaline pH
    b. neutral pH   d. no pH   ____

29. How can matter be changed?
    a. physically   c. physically and chemically
    b. chemically   d. cannot be changed   ____

30. In which form does matter exist?
    a. elements   c. mixtures
    b. compounds   d. all answers   ____

31. Quickly evaporating solutions are:
    a. weighty   c. volatile
    b. made up of isopropyl d. resolute
       alcohol   ____

32. Water, air, metals, and minerals are:
    a. elements   c. organic substances
    b. inorganic substances d. compounds   ____

33. Which of the following best describes matter?
    a. occupies space   c. exists as either a solid,
                               liquid, or gas
    b. has physical and   d. all answers
       chemical properties   ____

34. What are carbon, oxygen, nitrogen, silver, and sulfur?
    a. elements   c. compounds
    b. molecular substances d. all answers   ____

35. A pure substance:
    a. only has organic additives c. is unadulterated
    b. is a chemical combination   d. has a fixed chemical
       of matter, in definite   composition
       proportions   ____

CHAPTER 11—NAIL PRODUCT CHEMISTRY SIMPLIFIED

1. In order to accurately troubleshoot and solve common service breakdowns, you must have at least some basic knowledge of what?
   a. technical skills
   b. chemistry of your products
   c. ins-and-outs of a particular nail enhancement product
   d. experience _____

2. Are all odorless monomers vapor free?
   a. no
   b. yes
   c. depends on the brand
   d. only if the dappen dish is not designed properly _____

3. All the following are types of nail primer except:
   a. non-acid
   b. acid-free
   c. acid-base
   d. oil-based _____

4. What is the role of acetone in nail services?
   a. corrosive
   b. solvent
   c. adhesive
   d. solute _____

5. Define corrosive.
   a. material that can damage skin on contact
   b. acid-free primer with a neutral pH
   c. strong nail adhesive that causes two surfaces to stick together
   d. rust _____

6. What causes two surfaces to stick together?
   a. cross-linkers
   b. solutes
   c. adhesives
   d. solvents _____

7. What can you do to help avoid nail infections and lifting?
   a. scrubbing the hands and nails
   b. applying lots of primer
   c. roughing up the nail
   d. overfiling the natural nail _____

8. A _____ monomers can link together in less than 1 second.
   a. billion
   b. million
   c. trillion
   d. quadrillion _____

9. What is a common reason for enhancement breakdown?
   a. removing natural oils from the nail plate
   b. applying corrosives to the nail
   c. removing surface moisture
   d. over-filing _____

10. Define monomer.
    a. individual molecules that join together to make a polymer chain
    b. a chain nearly as large as a polymer chain
    c. clusters of molecules that join to make a polymer chain
    d. double chains of polymers   _____

11. Good adhesion begins with:
    a. corrosion   c. antibacterial spray
    b. clean, dry nails   d. buffed surface   _____

12. Monomers are cross linkers when they join different
    _____ together.
    a. initiators   c. histamines
    b. polymer chains   d. adhesives   _____

13. Which of the following are evaporation coatings?
    a. nail polish   c. base coat
    b. top coat   d. all answers   _____

14. What is the most common (and avoidable) skin condition suffered by nail technicians?
    a. psoriasis   c. pachyonychia
    b. tinea pedis   d. contact dermatitis   _____

15. How do nail polishes, top coats, and base coats harden?
    a. polymerization   c. through a chemical process
    b. different monomers   d. they are evaporation coatings _____

16. Any substance that is liquid at room temperature will form
    _____.
    a. fumes   c. primers
    b. vapors   d. coatings   _____

17. A(n) _____ is a substance that can cause visible and possibly permanent skin damage.
    a. adhesive   c. cross-linker
    b. initiator   d. corrosive   _____

18. The best thing clients can do for their natural nails is to:
    a. apply acrylic (methacrylate) artificial enhancements
    b. apply gel nails
    c. enlist the services of a skilled and educated nail technician
    d. apply nail strengtheners   _____

19. Everything you can see or touch except _____ and
    _____ is a chemical.
    a. light and electricity   c. acid and non-acid primers
    b. gas and vapors   d. catalysts and initiators   ____

20. How is toxicity determined?
    a. skin condition   c. overexposure
    b. time of year   d. general health   ____

21. Short chains of monomers that have had the growth of their
    chains halted before they become polymers are called:
    a. toxic   c. oligomers
    b. coatings   d. simple polymer chains   ____

22. It is important for nail technicians to have a basic
    understanding of chemistry because:
    a. they handle dangerous chemicals
    b. they could create explosive or corrosive situations
    c. they must constantly mix chemicals as part of their
       services
    d. almost everything they do depends on chemistry   ____

23. Products that cover the nail plate with a hard film are called:
    a. coating   c. primer
    b. dehydrator   d. oil   ____

24. _____ is a force of nature that makes two surfaces
    stick together.
    a. Molecules   c. Vapor
    b. Adhesion   d. Amino acid   ____

25. What are corrosive nail primers called?
    a. acid primers   c. non-acid primers
    b. acid-free primers   d. alkaline primers   ____

26. Corrosive acid-based primers can potentially:
    a. burn the nail bed   c. thin the nail plate
    b. damage the nail plate   d. all answers   ____

27. Which of the following aid(s) in good adhesion?
    a. proper technique   c. washing the hands and
                                       scrubbing the nail plate
    b. high-quality products   d. all answers   ____

28. With acid-free primers and non-acid primers:
    a. there are no known allergic reactions
    b. skin contact must be avoided
    c. acrylic nails are much easier to apply
    d. nails degrade easily   ____

29. What is the most common result of improper nail preparation?
    a. nail lifting   c. allergic reactions
    b. product breakdown   d. yellowing   _____

30. All nail enhancements form:
    a. vapors   c. infections
    b. noticeable odors   d. none of the choices
                                        available   _____

31. Nail products that improve artificial nail adhesion are called:
    a. base coat   c. sticky base coat
    b. primers   d. monomers   _____

32. Primers should be used:
    a. rarely   c. generously
    b. sparingly   d. every other time you
                                        perform a rebase service _____

33. You should always _____ any time you are having lifting
    problems.
    a. apply a second coat of primer
    b. review your application techniques and products
    c. make sure the client is not being careless at home
    d. decide that her nails are not a good candidate for artificial
       nail enhancements   _____

34. You should always dehydrate one hand at a time because:
    a. dust quickly settles on the nails
    b. bacteria quickly recolonize on natural nails
    c. oil and moisture return to the natural nail within 30 minutes
    d. dehydration can damage the nail plate   _____

35. Overfiling the nail plate creates a _____ for artificial nail
    enhancements.
    a. weaker foundation   c. more natural flexibility
    b. stronger foundation   d. more natural appearance _____

36. Overfiling (thinning) the nail plate causes what?
    a. free-edge product separations and breaking
    b. allergic reactions and infections under the nail plate
    c. painful friction burns and nail chipping
    d. all answers   _____

37. What causes poor nail adhesion?
    a. oil and moisture on the nail plate
    b. aggressive filing and improper application techniques
    c. poor-quality products
    d. all answers   _____

38. Identify two types of nail coatings.
   a. polish and acrylic (methacrylate) nail enhancements
   b. resins and nitrocellulose
   c. coatings that cure or polymerize; coatings that evaporate and harden
   d. hard and sticky   ____

39. Nail polishes and top coats undergo a:
   a. chemical reaction by evaporating and hardening
   b. physical reaction by hardening through evaporation
   c. chemical reaction through polymerization
   d. physical reaction by hardening through curing   ____

40. By undergoing a chemical process, acrylic (methacrylate) and UV gels:
   a. cure or polymerize   c. polymerize or monomer
   b. evaporate or harden   d. polymerize or evaporate   ____

41. Keratin is a(n):
   a. monomer   c. protein polymer
   b. polymer   d. amino acid   ____

42. What is polymerization?
   a. chemical reaction that bonds polymer molecules together to form a much larger molecule or monomer
   b. chemical reaction that bonds monomer molecules together to form a much larger molecule or polymer
   c. physical reaction that bonds polymer molecules together to form a much larger molecule or monomer
   d. physical reaction that bonds monomer molecules together to form a much larger molecule or polymer   ____

43. Polymerization causes:
   a. the product to thin   c. more room for the product
   b. thickening of the product   d. a shiny surface   ____

44. When a polymer chain's growth is halted before it is long enough to become a polymer, it is called a(n):
   a. multimonomer   c. minipolymer
   b. multimer   d. oligomer   ____

45. Oligomers are used for:
   a. rapid curing of gel nails   c. all nail enhancement services
   b. speeding up services when you are running behind   d. all answers   ____

46. The sticky surface on UV gels is caused by:
    a. oils   c. UV light
    b. oligomers   d. adhesion ingredient   _____

47. How do monomers attach to each other?
    a. head of one monomer   c. polymers to each other
       to the tail of another
    b. going tail to tail   d. amino acids together   _____

48. How are wraps and adhesives formed?
    a. simple monomer chains   c. helix coils
    b. simple polymer chains   d. cytokines   _____

49. You can unravel simple polymer chains used in wraps and
    adhesives by:
    a. blunt force   c. solvent
    b. heavy stress   d. all answers   _____

50. What do cross-linking agents do?
    a. strengthen monolithic   c. strengthen simple
       structures   polymer chains
    b. make wraps more brittle   d. keep adhesion to a
                                       minimum   _____

51. Cross-linking agents are like:
    a. a fishing net   c. wire mesh
    b. rungs of a ladder   d. a knitted fabric   _____

52. What do cross-linking agents do for natural and artificial nails?
    a. make them more durable   c. make them tougher and
                                       more resilient
    b. make them more resistant   d. all answers
       to solvents   _____

53. Define volatile solvent.
    a. one that is capable of pitting the nails
    b. one that evaporates quickly
    c. a solvent that produces no fumes
    d. an explosive solvent   _____

54. When base coats and top coats evaporate, what is left behind?
    a. only the color   c. durable color
    b. hardened polymer film   d. smooth surface   _____

55. Nail polishes _____ because they do not contain cross-linked polymers.
    a. are best suited for artificial nail enhancement products
    b. lose their luster
    c. smear easily
    d. chip easily
    ____

56. A toxic product is only bad or poisonous when:
    a. it is handled improperly   c. you touch it
    b. when you inhale the   d. it is consumed
       fumes
    ____

CHAPTER 12—BASICS OF ELECTRICITY

1. Define electricity.
    a. visible energy
    b. form of gas
    c. form of energy
    d. form of matter ____

2. Sparks and lightning are:
    a. flow of electrons
    b. effects of electricity
    c. negative charged particles
    d. shocking effects ____

3. Define electric current.
    a. flow of electricity along a conductor
    b. voltage
    c. conduit
    d. ampere ____

4. Which of the following best describes an insulator?
    a. complete circuit
    b. nonconductor
    c. twisted metal thread
    d. silk, wood, or glass ____

5. Any substance that _____ is considered to be a conductor.
    a. produces ions
    b. separates negatively charged electrons
    c. conducts ohms
    d. allows an electrical current to pass through it ____

6. An electric current will not flow through a conductor unless the force (volts) is stronger than the _____ or _____.
    a. amps, milliamps
    b. resistance, ohms
    c. watts, ohms
    d. current, force ____

7. All substances can be classified as:
    a. conductors and conduits
    b. having electrical properties
    c. conductors or insulators
    d. cord or cordless ____

8. What are electric wires?
    a. nonconductors
    b. generators
    c. insulators
    d. conductors ____

9. Why should you never swim in a lake during a lightning storm?
    a. Water contains no ions.
    b. Lake water has a high metallic content.
    c. This is an urban myth.
    d. Ions in water are good conductors of electricity. ____

10. When a current flows in only one direction, it is called a:
    a. direct current
    b. alternating current
    c. straight current
    d. one-way current ____

11. Which of the following is (are) true about alternating current?
    a. It flows in one direction and then the other.
    b. It changes direction 60 times a second.
    c. Any appliance that plugs into the wall uses alternating current.
    d. All answers.
    ____

12. Water molecules flow through a hose like:
    a. electrons flow through a wire
    b. electrons flow through glass
    c. electricity flows through the atmosphere
    d. all answers
    ____

13. What makes electrons flow?
    a. volts
    b. pressure
    c. amperes
    d. watts
    ____

14. What kind of electrical current powers flashlights, cellular telephones, and cordless electric files?
    a. alternating current
    b. batteries
    c. direct current
    d. no current of any kind
    ____

15. What is a converter?
    a. regulates the amount of electrical output
    b. transforms direct current into alternating current
    c. does not exist
    d. allows you to control the amount of watts per second
    ____

16. How many watts per second will a 40-watt lightbulb use?
    a. 4
    b. 40
    c. 400
    d. 4,000
    ____

17. Which of the following reveals the number of watts in a kilowatt?
    a. 100 watts
    b. 1,000 watts
    c. 10,000 watts
    d. 1,000,000 watts
    ____

18. A 1,000-watt (1-kilowatt) hair dryer uses:
    a. 1,000 watts of energy per second
    b. 1,000 watts of energy per minute
    c. 10,000 watts of energy per second
    d. 10,000 watts of energy per minute
    ____

19. What type of substance makes reactions happen quicker?
    a. light
    b. catalyst
    c. heat
    d. water
    ____

20. What is the role of a catalyst?
    a. act like initiators
    c. absorb energy like a battery
    b. emit ultraviolet rays
    d. shield the product from sunlight
    ____

21. UV-light cured enhancements use UV light to produce:
    a. physical effects
    c. chemical effects and kill germs
    b. chemical effects
    d. ultraviolet (UV light)
    ____

22. To ensure that your electrical equipment is in good working order, how often should it be inspected?
    a. when you first take it out of the box
    c. never
    b. during your annual inspection
    d. regularly
    ____

23. Careless electrical connections and overloaded circuits can result in a(n):
    a. burn
    c. electrical shock
    b. serious fire
    d. all answers
    ____

24. A fuse or breaker does what?
    a. prevents excessive current from passing through a circuit
    b. prevents excessive current from passing through a wire
    c. maintains a steady flow of electricity
    d. minimizes fires
    ____

25. A unit that measures the pressure or force that pushes the flow of electrons forward through a conductor is called a:
    a. watt
    c. volt
    b. amp
    d. kilowatt
    ____

26. What is the difference between a fuse and a circuit breaker?
    a. One is a switch, one blows out or melts.
    c. There is no difference.
    b. They both blow out and melt.
    d. A fuse is a true switch.
    ____

27. What have modern circuit breakers replaced?
    a. silk-wrapped wires
    c. electrical light switches
    b. fuses
    d. outlets
    ____

28. When a circuit breaker pops or turns off, what should you do before resetting?
    a. turn off the appliances
    c. check all connections
    b. inspect insulation
    d. all answers
    ____

29. What is the purpose of the Underwriter's Laboratory (UL) certification?
    a. It rates the number of hours appliances can be safely used before switching off.
    b. It certifies the safety of electrical appliances.
    c. It informs you of the type and number of circuit breakers needed to safely use the appliance.
    d. It is only used when appliances use more than 1,000 watts of power.   _____

30. What symbol should you look for on appliances before purchasing?
    a. manufacturer's symbol of safety   c. number of watts
    b. manufacturer's instruction manual   d. Underwriter's Laboratory (UL) symbol   _____

31. What is a ground connection?
    a. connection that is buried in the ground
    b. a slightly larger prong
    c. connection that completes the circuit and carries the current safely away to the ground
    d. added protection   _____

32. Identify the most important advantage of having an extra ground.
    a. It protects you if the first ground fails.
    b. It protects you by splitting the electricity into two paths.
    c. It prevents shocks.
    d. It allows the appliances to work for longer periods of time without overheating.   _____

33. When you are through using an electrical appliance, you should:
    a. turn it off and unplug it   c. make sure it is upright
    b. turn it off   d. flip the circuit breaker   _____

34. How should you disconnect appliances?
    a. pulling on the cord   c. pulling on the appliance
    b. pulling on the plug   d. none of the choices available   _____

35. When electrical cords become twisted, it could cause:
    a. an inconvenient situation   c. wires to go haywire.
    b. a short circuit   d. wires to ground each other   _____

36. You should avoid contact with water and metal surfaces when using electricity because:
    a. water and metal are conductors
    b. electricity is attracted to water and metal
    c. there is a potential for shock
    d. all answers

    ____

37. You should never place objects on or _____ electric cords.
    a. step over
    b. step on
    c. hide
    d. near

    ____

38. The only time you should attempt to repair an electrical appliance is if:
    a. you are qualified and certified
    b. it is a simple job
    c. you think you know what you are doing
    d. there is no one around to help you

    ____

CHAPTER 13—MANICURING

1. Which of the following condition(s) would benefit from a conditioning oil manicure?
    a. brittle nails
    b. nail ridges
    c. dry skin around the nail plate
    d. all answers
    _____

2. Define paraffin.
    a. a petroleum by-product
    b. a jellylike substance
    c. an organic oil
    d. a non-petroleum form of wax
    _____

3. In men's manicures, what replaces the colored polish step?
    a. 30-minute massage
    b. matte top coat or buffing service
    c. callus removal
    d. hand softening treatment
    _____

4. What are the contraindications for a paraffin wax treatment?
    a. sensitivities to heat due to medications or thinning skin
    b. skin irritations
    c. impaired circulation
    d. all answers
    _____

5. Hand-and-arm massage is always done as part of:
    a. a spa manicure
    b. a manicure service when clients are stressed
    c. a slower period of the day
    d. when the timing seems right
    _____

6. Define effleurage.
    a. rolling and kneading
    b. wringing movements
    c. rapid tapping movements
    d. long, smooth strokes
    _____

7. When should the massage portion of the manicure be done?
    a. after the manicure, and before the polish
    b. at the beginning, and before the client pays
    c. at the beginning, and after the cuticle remover is applied
    d. any time
    _____

8. Special units utilized to melt solid wax into liquid should be maintained generally at what temperature?
    a. 125°F to 130°F
    b. 25°F to 30°F
    c. 200°F to 300°F
    d. 76°F to 80°F
    _____

9. You can practice sound ergonomics while massaging your clients' hands and feet by:
    a. keeping your legs straight
    b. keeping your shoulders level
    c. standing up
    d. never leaning toward your client
    _____

10. What medical condition(s) are contraindicative of massage?
   a. heart condition
   c. clients who have had, or are at risk for, a stroke
   b. high blood pressure
   d. all answers

   _____

11. Define aromatherapy.
   a. the medical science of well-being
   b. botanical essential oils used to promote a sense of well-being
   c. a new-age solution to stress
   d. moisturizing oils that deeply penetrate the skin

   _____

12. A _____ is applied over colored polish to prevent chipping and to add a shine to the finished nail.
   a. base coat
   c. gel
   b. top coat
   d. acrylic

   _____

13. Colored coatings applied to the natural nail plate are also known as:
   a. enamel
   c. varnish
   b. lacquer
   d. all answers

   _____

14. To prevent a yellowish staining or other discoloration to the natural nail plate, apply a _____ before colored polish.
   a. coat of gel
   c. resin
   b. base coat
   d. polish dryer

   _____

15. Define massage.
   a. kneading and stroking
   b. manipulating the body through a series of specific movements
   c. percussion
   d. tapping and wringing

   _____

16. Nail conditioners contain ingredients to reduce _____ of the nail plate and moisturize the surrounding skin.
   a. redness
   c. swelling
   b. brittleness
   d. infections

   _____

17. Most things that are used once on clients and then discarded are called:
   a. equipment
   c. materials or supplies
   b. implements
   d. cosmetics

   _____

18. Identify the implement(s) that are disposable:
   a. acetone
   c. wooden pusher
   b. nail polish
   d. cotton

   _____

19. The recommended wattage for a bulb used in a manicure lamp is between _____ watts.
   a. 25 and 30
   b. 30 and 35
   c. 40 and 60
   d. 60 and 75 _____

20. Implements that must be sanitized and disinfected before each client include:
   a. nail clippers
   b. tweezers
   c. metal pushers
   d. all answers _____

21. Metal implements must be _____ before being disinfected.
   a. cleaned with a towel
   b. washed with soap and water
   c. cleaned in an autoclave
   d. rinsed in alcohol _____

22. Use a(n) _____ to shape the free edge.
   a. wooden pusher
   b. abrasive file
   c. metal pusher
   d. tweezers _____

23. What should you do with an implement that has been used on a client?
   a. rinse with water
   b. wipe off with cotton
   c. bag and discard
   d. clean and disinfect _____

24. To remove nail cosmetics from their containers, use a:
   a. wooden pusher
   b. metal pusher
   c. plastic or metal spatula
   d. cotton swab _____

25. Identify the proper way to immerse implements in a disinfectant solution.
   a. wipe thoroughly
   b. quickly rinse
   c. fully immerse
   d. dip slightly _____

26. Nail clippers are beneficial when shortening the nail length because they:
   a. create a high shine
   b. reduce filing time
   c. strengthen weak nails
   d. reduce splitting _____

27. The best implement for smoothing out wavy ridges and creating a shiny nail plate is a:
   a. nail clipper
   b. ridge filler
   c. abrasive file
   d. three-way buffer _____

28. The rule of thumb is the lower the grit, the larger the abrasive particles on the board and the _____ its action
   a. softer
   b. swifter
   c. finer
   d. more aggressive _____

29. What is the best way to prevent excessive odors and control vapors from nail services in salons?
    a. plastic trash can
    b. multiple paper bags
    c. ventilated receptacles with lids
    d. metal receptacle with self-closing lid
    _____

30. Before applying base coat, you must:
    a. apply cuticle remover
    b. soak the fingers in a finger bowl
    c. remove all traces of oil
    d. wash hands thoroughly
    _____

31. A _____ is used to clean fingernails and remove debris.
    a. nail file
    b. chamois buffer
    c. wooden pusher
    d. nail brush
    _____

32. A _____ is used to soften cuticles and increase the flexibility of natural nails.
    a. cuticle remover
    b. polish remover
    c. penetrating oil
    d. nail bleach
    _____

33. Key ingredients in nail hardener formulations include nylon, protein, and:
    a. UV gels
    b. formaldehyde
    c. potassium hydroxide
    d. acetone
    _____

34. Quick-dry nail polish products may be sprayed on or applied with a:
    a. wooden pusher
    b. metal pusher
    c. cotton swab
    d. dropper
    _____

35. When the free edge has no rounding at the edges and is filed straight across, it is called:
    a. pointed
    b. round
    c. square
    d. squoval
    _____

36. When the nail extends slightly past the fingertip and is shaped in a gentle c-curve, it is called:
    a. round
    b. pointed
    c. squoval
    d. square
    _____

37. A top coat or sealer makes nail polish:
    a. dry more quickly
    b. adhere to nail plate
    c. resistant to chipping
    d. bubble free
    _____

38. Manicures consist of these three parts or segments:
    a. pre-service, service, post-service
    b. actual service, post-service, follow-up
    c. pre-service, post-service, follow-up
    d. pre-service, post-service, product recommendation ____

39. A polish design that has a dramatic _____ on the free edge is called a French manicure.
    a. peach   c. white
    b. pink   d. neutral ____

CHAPTER 14—PEDICURING

1. How often should a client have a pedicure to ensure healthy, happy feet?
   - a. weekly
   - b. daily
   - c. yearly
   - d. monthly ____

2. When clients come to their pedicure appointments wearing closed-toed shoes, what should you have them wear afterwards to prevent the polish from being marred or smeared?
   - a. toenail clippers
   - b. pedicure slippers
   - c. toe separators
   - d. pedicure footrest ____

3. For your convenience, a pedicure station should be near what?
   - a. sink
   - b. front door
   - c. waiting area
   - d. lounge ____

4. Pedicures are particularly important to which of the following?
   - a. joggers
   - b. dancers
   - c. cosmetologists
   - d. all answers ____

5. What is the ideal way to clip the toenails when performing a pedicure?
   - a. extremely short
   - b. long and elegant
   - c. pointed and thinned
   - d. even with end of toe ____

6. What is an important part of a pedicure post-service procedure?
   - a. compliment the client
   - b. advise the client
   - c. help the client exit quickly
   - d. soothe the client ____

7. What is the name for a fully-plumbed, free-standing pedicure unit?
   - a. pedicure throne
   - b. wet chair
   - c. royal chair
   - d. whirlpool unit ____

8. What is a rasp?
   - a. a nail file
   - b. a file used most often used for the sides of the big toe
   - c. a big toe separator
   - d. a multidirectional tool ____

9. When massaging the feet and calves, a light or hard stroking movement is called:
   - a. effleurage
   - b. petrissage
   - c. tapotement
   - d. percussion ____

10. To properly clean and disinfect your pedicure tub as directed by your state regulations, a minimum would be:
    a. after each use
    b. at the end of each week
    c. at the end of each day
    d. at the end of each month ____

11. In massage, a movement that includes kneading, squeezing, and friction is called:
    a. effleurage
    b. percussion
    c. petrissage
    d. tapotement ____

12. Clients with poor circulation or diabetes must _____ before having a pedicure service.
    a. sign a liability release form
    b. provide a doctor's release
    c. read a pamphlet covering the risks of having a pedicure service
    d. give verbal consent to proceed with service ____

13. The products used in a pedicure bath to soften the skin are called:
    a. foot soaks
    b. foot rubs
    c. foot scrubs
    d. foot masques ____

14. What type of product is used to soften cuticles for removal from the nail plate?
    a. cuticle strengtheners
    b. nail plate dissolvers
    c. cuticle softeners
    d. cuticle removers ____

15. What is the name of the implement with an end that is shaped like an ice cream scoop?
    a. rasp
    b. nail scoop
    c. curette
    d. metal pusher ____

16. A light or hard stroking massage movement that relaxes muscles and improves circulation is called:
    a. petrissage
    b. effleurage
    c. tapotement
    d. friction ____

17. What products are used to smooth dry, flaky skin and calluses?
    a. massage preparations
    b. scrubs
    c. sea salts
    d. clay masques ____

18. In foot massage, the metatarsal scissors technique is a _____ movement.
    a. percussion
    b. effleurage
    c. petrissage
    d. tapotement ____

19. An implement designed to file in one direction is called:
    a. curette
    c. a rasp
    b. foot file
    d. clipper
    _____

20. What does it mean to exfoliate the skin?
    a. remove dead, dry skin
    c. remove the stratum corneum
    b. remove the first layer of skin
    d. rub the skin with a thick oil
    _____

21. What is the purpose of a callus softener?
    a. soften and strengthen calluses, especially on heels and over pressure points
    b. soften and smooth calluses, especially on heels and over pressure points
    c. dissolve skin
    d. remove corns and calluses
    _____

22. What is a foot file used for?
    a. to smooth calluses and remove dry, flaky skin
    b. to paddle the soles of the feet as part of a percussion massage
    c. to smooth skin on the hands and feet
    d. to shape the toenails
    _____

23. Why should a callus never be removed?
    a. A callus is a protective covering.
    b. It should be removed only by a podiatrist.
    c. It should be dissolved, not manually removed.
    d. Callus protects the bones.
    _____

24. What are nippers used for?
    a. to remove dead skin on the heel
    b. to trim the nail
    c. to remove dead tags of skin around the nail plate
    d. to remove one layer of living tissue
    _____

25. Which of the following are characteristics of a cuticle remover?
    a. highly alkaline, corrosive, and fast acting
    c. highly acidic, noncorrosive, and fast acting
    b. highly acidic, corrosive, and fast acting
    d. highly alkaline, noncorrosive, and fast acting
    _____

CHAPTER 15—ELECTRIC FILING

1. Define torque.
   a. amount of motor resistance
   b. RPMs
   c. power of machine's motor
   d. shank size _____

2. Which of these machines is recommended for professional nail technicians?
   a. micromotor
   b. belt-driven
   c. macromotor
   d. portable drills _____

3. Rings of fire are caused by:
   a. filing too aggressively
   b. motor running too slowly
   c. coarse abrasives
   d. improper angle of bit _____

4. What denotes the speed of an electric file?
   a. miles per hour (MPH)
   b. revolutions per minute (RPM)
   c. nanoturns
   d. high, medium, and low _____

5. Concentric bits are important because they:
   a. do not wobble
   b. do not heat up as quickly
   c. are easier to attach
   d. produce better results _____

6. When bits have sharp edges, they should be:
   a. smoothed with a 240 grit abrasive
   b. filed while bit is spinning at low speed
   c. returned to manufacturer
   d. used until edges become dull _____

7. Sander, diamond, _____, and _____, are the four most common types of bits used by salon professionals.
   a. carbide, Swiss carbide
   b. tourmaline, ruby
   c. buffers, filers
   d. flutes, sleeves _____

8. The particles produced by sanders or sleeves (bits):
   a. require frequent sanitizing of surfaces
   b. float high and are easily inhaled
   c. do not pose a health risk
   d. are healthier to use than metal bits _____

9. Carbide bits are unique because they:
   a. have flutes instead of grit
   b. last the longest
   c. are disposable
   d. are the least expensive _____

10. An electric file that has a forward-and-reverse feature is important when:
    a. you are right-handed
    b. you are an expert
    c. you are left-handed
    d. you suffer from wrist fatigue _____

11. The ruby or sapphire particles on pedicure bits are commonly used to:
   a. smooth corns
   b. smooth calluses
   c. remove imbedded dirt
   d. all answers
   _____

12. It is important to keep the bit _____ when using an electric file.
   a. perpendicular to the table
   b. flat with wrist turned slight downward
   c. flat and parallel with the table
   d. flat and parallel to your shoulders
   _____

13. Under the free edge, barrel-shaped or tapered Swiss carbide bits are best for:
   a. refining c-curves
   b. making a perfect squoval
   c. squaring nail tips
   d. u-shaped surfaces
   _____

14. To ensure that an artificial nail enhancement has no visible scratches, you should finish the nail by:
   a. using nail oil
   b. using cream and pumice powder
   c. graduating bits coarse to fine
   d. finishing with a buffer bit
   _____

15. Grabbing can avoided by:
   a. keeping the bit parallel to the table
   b. angling the finger, not the bit
   c. using bits with rounded ends
   d. all answers
   _____

16. Which of the following describe(s) potential causes of microshattering?
   a. using poor-quality bits
   b. handpiece held at wrong angle
   c. working too aggressively
   d. all answers
   _____

17. Vibration can cause:
   a. nail tips to crack
   b. damage to fingertips
   c. carpal tunnel syndrome
   d. excessive nervousness
   _____

18. How do you disinfect a metal bit?
   a. You do not; they are disposable.
   b. Disinfect by hand to avoid damage.
   c. Disinfect the same way as any nondisposable implement.
   d. Disinfect while the bit is running.
   _____

19. What does AEFM stand for?
    a. Association of Electric File Manufacturers
    b. Association of Eclectic File Manufacturers
    c. Association of Ergonomic File Manufacturers
    d. Association of Egregious File Manufacturers   ____

20. Why is the AEFM important to nail technicians?
    a. It is a training organization. c. It is product-neutral.
    b. It sets safety standards   d. All answers.
       for the nail industry.   ____

21. An electric file with a closed casing can prolong the life of your
    machine because:
    a. it is more comfortable to hold
    b. it keeps dust out of the casing and the internal
       mechanisms
    c. it is a more expensive machine
    d. it prevents air from blowing on your client's hands while
       working   ____

22. Why is a keyless feature beneficial to nail technicians?
    a. You can change bits with one hand.
    b. It allows you to use many different kinds of bits.
    c. You do not have to worry about losing your key.
    d. It makes it easier to change bits.   ____

23. Machines with smaller motors and lighter handpieces have:
    a. a better design   c. less power
    b. the same amount of   d. no power
       power   ____

24. A micromotor machine has a motor that is so small:
    a. it is electric   c. it weighs only 5 ounces
    b. the motor barely vibrates   d. it is housed in the
                                        handpiece   ____

25. Two things can cause bits to rust:
    a. poor quality and soaking too long in disinfectant
    b. cuticle softener and cuticle remover
    c. polish and polish remover
    d. oils and lotions   ____

26. When using sanders or sleeves, the greatest disadvantage is
    that:
    a. they wear out mid-service c. they tend to grab the nail
    b. dust particles float in the d. they overheat
       air and can be inhaled   ____

27. Diamond bits that are lower quality:
    a. are less versatile than sanders
    b. may cause scratches on the surface of the nail
    c. tend to skip
    d. are only available in one grit   ____

28. Traditional carbide bits:
    a. will skip on the return stroke leaving scratches on the surface of the enhancement
    b. are the same as cross-cut carbide bits
    c. are the same as Swiss carbide bits
    d. are made out of an inferior alloy when compared to Swiss carbide bits   ____

29. Some of the characteristics of higher-quality diamond bits are:
    a. Construction is more consistent because each particle on every bit is cut the same size and shape and then adhered to a medical stainless steel bit.
    b. Seventy percent of the particles are higher-quality diamonds.
    c. Each diamond chip is hand assembled on a medical-grade stainless steel metal bit.
    d. All diamond chips come from the same stone.   ____

30. When filing the sides of the nail, which bit should you use?
    a. cross-cut carbide bit
    b. Swiss carbide bit
    c. sander or sleeve
    d. ruby   ____

31. Describe buffing bits:
    a. bits made of soft materials like chamois, leather, or goat's hair
    b. bits made of very fine particles
    c. disposable cloth bits
    d. three-way bits   ____

32. What is the most important benefit of using higher speeds with your electric file?
    a. doing a better job
    b. working faster
    c. applying less pressure
    d. working equally well on gels and acrylics (methacrylate)   ____

33. To smooth old product in the regrowth area of the nail, prep this area with a:
    a. fine-grit bit
    b. medium-grit bit
    c. Swiss carbide bit
    d. only a diamond bit   ____

34. Why are buffing oils frequently used when using an electric file?
    a. They condition the cuticles.
    b. They reduce heat and hold dust on the surface of the bit.
    c. They create a glossy shine.
    d. They enhance smoothness of UV gels if used before applying UV gel sealers.   ____

35. Which bits create the least amount of airborne dust?
    a. sanders and sleeves   c. carbide and Swiss carbide bits
    b. diamond bits   d. pedicure bits   ____

36. Any time you find yourself feeling the need to press harder on the nail, you should:
    a. press harder   c. be more patient
    b. reduce speed   d. increase speed   ____

CHAPTER 16—NAIL TIPS, WRAPS, AND NO-LIGHT GELS

1. An artificial nail tip is made from what material?
    a. common plastic used to make utensils
    b. tenite acetate polymer or ABS
    c. monomer and polymer
    d. ceramic   _____

2. An artificial nail product that is used to add length is called a(n):
    a. overlay   c. nail wrap
    b. acrylic nail   d. nail tip   _____

3. What is the primary purpose of a nail tip?
    a. repair a damaged nail   c. overlay for gels
    b. add length to nail   d. overlay for acrylic
                                   (methacrylate) nail
                                   enhancements   _____

4. In order for a nail tip to be durable, it must be reinforced with a(n):
    a. well   c. adhesive
    b. resin activator   d. overlay   _____

5. When applying a nail tip, an abrasive is used to:
    a. attach the tip   c. remove the tip
    b. attach the wrap   d. remove surface shine _____

6. The _____ is the point of contact with the nail plate.
    a. nail tip   c. nail wrap
    b. nail well   d. nail resin   _____

7. What should you wear when handling nail adhesive?
    a. face shield   c. safety eyewear
    b. gloves   d. nonabsorbent apron   _____

8. A nail tip should cover no more than _____ of the natural nail.
    a. 1/4   c. 1/16
    b. 1/3   d. 1/8   _____

9. Nail tips have a shallow depression called a:
    a. free edge   c. well
    b. plate   d. dip   _____

10. You apply a nail tip to the nail plate by using:
   a. the stop, rock, and hold procedure
   b. a cotton-tipped wooden pusher
   c. a small nail brush
   d. the stop, rock, and slide procedure ____

11. To create the least amount of damage to the natural nail, you should remove softened nail tips by:
   a. rubbing them off   c. sliding them off
   b. pulling them off   d. nipping them off ____

12. A thin, elongated board with a rough surface is called a(n):
   a. abrasive   c. buffer
   b. nipper   d. adhesive ____

13. When you bond nail-size pieces of cloth or paper to the top of the nail plate, what service are you performing?
   a. repair patch   c. nail wrap
   b. UV gel   d. buffer wrap ____

14. Using a piece of fabric cut to precisely cover a crack in the nail is called a:
   a. nail wrap   c. no-light gel
   b. repair patch   d. fiberglass resin ____

15. Which nail wrapping material becomes transparent when adhesive is applied?
   a. silk   c. satin
   b. linen   d. cotton ____

16. You can cut nail tips with a special implement called a:
   a. nail clipper   c. nail nipper
   b. nail cutter   d. tip cutter ____

17. Acrylic (methacrylate) liquid and powder, wraps, or UV gels are used as _____ on natural nails.
   a. nail tips   c. underlays
   b. overlays   d. wraps ____

18. The thickness of adhesive is called:
   a. oil remover   c. viscosity
   b. dehydrator   d. polymer ____

19. The product that is designed to remove moisture from the nail plate is called:
   a. a dehydrator   c. soap and water
   b. polish thinner   d. cuticle remover ____

20. You can minimize damage to the natural nail when applying nail tips by:
    a. buffing the nail wrap
    b. using a fine abrasive
    c. applying resin activator
    d. preblending the nail tip _____

21. To harden no-light gels, a small amount of _____ is dispensed atop of the enhancement.
    a. resin
    b. oil
    c. activator
    d. gel _____

22. A perfect nail tip fit:
    a. is the perfect shape
    b. covers the nail plate from sidewall to sidewall
    c. means the tip covers the entire nail perfectly
    d. means the tip is not too long _____

23. When you do not have a tip that perfectly fits your client's nail, you should:
    a. glue two tips together
    b. use a larger one and file it down to size
    c. find the closest one that fits
    d. refuse the service _____

24. In the stop, rock, and hold method of applying tips, the tip should be held:
    a. with tweezers
    b. at a 45-degree angle
    c. at a 90-degree angle
    d. with your pinkie _____

25. The _____ motion is the second step of a nail tip application.
    a. rock
    b. roll
    c. jiggle
    d. freeze _____

26. The third step of a nail tip application is to _____ the tip in place.
    a. hold
    b. do not hold
    c. squeeze
    d. press _____

27. Identify the safest way(s) to remove a fabric nail wrap.
    a. Soak the nail wrap in an acetone solution until softened.
    b. Slide off the nail wrap using a wooden pusher.
    c. Buff the nail to remove any adhesive residue.
    d. All answers. _____

28. What is a nail wrap used for?
    a. to correct spoon-shaped nails
    b. to keep the natural nails in tip-top shape
    c. to lengthen nails
    d. less expensive way to have long beautiful nails _____

29. How should you apply fabric adhesive when using a non-adhesive backed fabric?
    a. a thin line down the center of the nail
    b. one drop in the center of the nail plate
    c. over the entire nail
    d. only on the nail tip

    _____

30. A wrap resin should be applied:
    a. down the center of the nail with an extender tip
    b. all over the nail wrap
    c. a drop in the center of the nail
    d. in a crisscross fashion using a nail extender tip

    _____

31. Between the fabric and the sidewalls, you should leave _____ margin.
    a. a 1/16-inch   c. a 1/8-inch
    b. a 1/32-inch   d. no

    _____

32. Allowing nail adhesive to extend from the nail wrap to the skin can cause:
    a. skin irritation and nail pitting
    b. skin irritation and loose cuticles
    c. skin irritation and lifting
    d. lifting and damaged matrix

    _____

33. You should maintain fabric wraps every:
    a. 1 week   c. month
    b. 2 weeks   d. 6 weeks

    _____

34. Using an activator with fabric wraps:
    a. makes the wrap stick to the nail plate
    b. makes the fabric more durable
    c. shortens the amount of time it takes to wrap the nails
    d. speeds up the hardening process

    _____

35. The protocol for a two-week maintenance appointment of fabric wraps involves:
    a. applying wrap resin to new nail growth only
    b. applying accelerator to the entire nail
    c. applying a fresh coat of wrap resin to the entire nail
    d. all answers

    _____

CHAPTER 17—ACRYLIC (METHACRYLATE) NAIL ENHANCEMENTS

1. Artificial nail enhancements that use a liquid-and-powder system are made of:
   a. acrylic (methacrylate)   c. synthetics
   b. polycrylic   d. monocrylic   ____

2. The technical name for the subcategory of acrylic substances that is used to make nail enhancements is called:
   a. acrylate   c. methacrylic
   b. methacrylate   d. polyacrylics   ____

3. Acrylic nails are a _____-and-powder system.
   a. primer   c. adhesive
   b. liquid   d. powder   ____

4. The polymer in acrylic nail enhancements is in the:
   a. powder   c. liquid
   b. dehydrator   d. adhesive   ____

5. A monomer unit is made up of one:
   a. primer   c. catalyst
   b. initiator   d. molecule   ____

6. The monomer liquid portion of acrylic nails consists of which substance?
   a. isopropyl methacrylate   c. methacrylate
   b. benzoyl peroxide   d. ethyl alcohol   ____

7. Acrylic (methacrylate) nail enhancements are hardened by a chemical process called:
   a. rebalancing   c. molecular hardening
   b. polymerization   d. initiation   ____

8. Surface moisture is removed from the nails prior to an acrylic (methacrylate) service by using a:
   a. dehydrator   c. primer
   b. initiator   d. catalyst   ____

9. The chemical reaction is accelerated by using a(n):
   a. dehydrator   c. primer
   b. catalyst   d. initiator   ____

10. The catalyst energizes and activates the:
    a. initiator   c. primer
    b. dehydrator   d. gel   ____

11. Which product is used to ensure strong adhesion and prevent lifting problems with acrylic (methacrylate) nails?
   a. dehydrator
   b. initiator
   c. primer
   d. catalyst
   _____

12. A polymer chain is created by a _____ that causes monomers to chemically link together.
   a. rebalancing
   b. molecular reaction
   c. chain reaction
   d. initiator reaction
   _____

13. The set or cure time is controlled by catalysts that are added to the:
   a. adhesive
   b. catalyst
   c. powder
   d. liquid
   _____

14. Benzoyl peroxide is a(n) _____ that is added to the powder to start a chain reaction that leads to long polymer chains.
   a. initiator
   b. catalyst
   c. dehydrator
   d. primer
   _____

15. When you use the wrong powder with your chosen liquid, your artificial nail enhancements could be:
   a. too brittle
   b. too flimsy
   c. improperly cured
   d. all answers
   _____

16. The amount of liquid and powder used to create an acrylic bead is called the:
   a. wet bead
   b. dry bead
   c. medium bead
   d. mix ratio
   _____

17. Which mix ratio is needed to create a medium bead?
   a. 50% more liquid than powder
   b. equal parts
   c. 50% more powder than liquid
   d. 3/4 liquid to 1/4 powder
   _____

18. An acrylic bead is created by doing what?
   a. mixing powder and liquid
   b. dipping brush in liquid, then in powder
   c. dipping brush in powder, then in liquid
   d. combining liquid and powder in a dappen dish
   _____

19. The three types of bead mix ratios are:
   a. wet, medium, dry
   b. thin, medium, thick
   c. loose, medium, set
   d. runny, medium, hard
   _____

20. The ideal mix ratio for working with monomer liquids and polymer powders:
    a. is generally dry   c. is generally wet
    b. is generally medium   d. depends on the type of enhancement you are forming   ____

21. You must use the correct mixture of powder and liquid in order to ensure the proper set and maximum _____ of the nail enhancement.
    a. resiliency   c. adaptability
    b. durability   d. beauty   ____

22. If too little powder is used, a nail enhancement can be:
    a. discolored   c. rubbery
    b. too strong   d. weak   ____

23. A(n) _____ primer is corrosive to the skin and potentially dangerous to the eyes.
    a. alkaline-based   c. monomer-based
    b. acid-based   d. alcohol-based   ____

24. Dappen dishes must have a narrow opening to:
    a. minimize evaporation   c. minimize condensation
    b. maximize evaporation   d. maximize condensation   ____

25. When applying acrylic nail enhancements, the best brush bristle is made of:
    a. sable hair   c. mink hair
    b. synthetic fiber   d. bristle fiber   ____

26. _____ gloves work best for nail-related applications.
    a. Nitrile polyester   c. Benzoyl polymer
    b. Nitrile polymer   d. Benzoyl polyester   ____

27. When tapped with the end of your brush, acrylic nail enhancements will make a clicking sound when they are hard enough to:
    a. nip and trim   c. clip and trim
    b. polish and finish   d. file and shape   ____

28. Nail enhancements that are not properly maintained have a greater tendency to:
    a. grow and strengthen   c. grow slower
    b. lift and break   d. split and chip   ____

29. The beauty, durability, and longevity of an artificial nail enhancement are achieved through this maintenance service:
    a. refreshing
    c. rebalancing
    b. servicing
    d. restructuring
    _____

30. You can cause lifting problems and possible damage to the _____ by nipping off acrylic material, whether it is loose or attached to the nail.
    a. nail bed
    c. nail plate
    b. hyponychium
    d. matrix
    _____

31. Odorless acrylic (methacrylate) nail enhancement products harden more slowly and form a(n) _____ layer on top of the nail.
    a. exhibition
    c. inhibition
    b. sticky
    d. assertion
    _____

32. Which motion is required to create the proper mix of powder and liquid with low-odor acrylic (methacrylate) products?
    a. multiple circular motions
    c. multiple vertical dipping motions
    b. single dip
    d. minimal circular motions
    _____

33. Low-odor products generally require which type of bead mix ratio?
    a. dry
    c. medium
    b. wet
    d. hard
    _____

34. Odorless acrylic products have the same chemical composition as regular acrylic products except they rely on _____ that have little odor.
    a. monomers
    c. acid primers
    b. polymers
    d. catalysts
    _____

35. The addition of product to repair an enhancement is called:
    a. fill-in
    c. stress strip
    b. rebalancing
    d. crack repair
    _____

36. You should _____ when filing away the inhibition layer of a low-odor acrylic product.
    a. wear a mask
    b. avoid contact with the freshly filed particles
    c. use a disposable file
    d. never file away these particles.
    _____

37. A basic way to apply liquid and powder products is:
    a. as a protective overlay
    c. sculpted using a flexible form
    b. over a nail tip
    d. all answers
    _____

CHAPTER 18—UV GELS

1. UV gel enhancements rely on what family of ingredients?
    - a. wrap resin
    - b. adhesives
    - c. fiberglass
    - d. acrylic

    _____

2. Which ingredients in UV gels cut the curing time from 3 hours to 3 minutes?
    - a. monomers
    - b. oligomers
    - c. polymers
    - d. primers

    _____

3. What sets UV gel nail enhancements apart from all other nail enhancements?
    - a. soaking
    - b. clipping
    - c. filing
    - d. curing

    _____

4. Urethane acrylate and urethane methacrylate are responsible for making what?
    - a. fiberglass wraps
    - b. UV gels
    - c. sculptured nails
    - d. nail tips

    _____

5. How do you measure the amount of electricity that UV bulbs consume?
    - a. voltages
    - b. amperes
    - c. ohms
    - d. wattage

    _____

6. What applicator is used to spread UV gel product onto the nail?
    - a. synthetic brushes
    - b. natural brushes
    - c. wooden pushers
    - d. metal pushers

    _____

7. Adhesion of UV gels to the natural nail plate is enhanced by using this product:
    - a. UV gel glue
    - b. UV gel primer
    - c. UV gel paste
    - d. UV gel buffer

    _____

8. What is the proper term for dipping the tip of the applicator brush into nail primer to ensure that the nail plate is covered?
    - a. priming the tip
    - b. dehydrating the eponychium
    - c. natural nail preparation
    - d. conditioning the nail

    _____

9. UV gel #1 is referred to as the:
    - a. base coat gel
    - b. primer coat gel
    - c. builder gel
    - d. sealer gel

    _____

10. The tacky surface layer of a UV gel nail enhancement is called the _____ layer.
    a. contour   c. aggressive
    b. integumentary   d. inhibition   _____

11. When contouring a UV gel nail, what grit should you be using?
    a. coarse   c. very fine
    b. medium   d. metal   _____

12. What happens when you expose your UV gel product to sunlight, full-spectrum manicure light, or UV gel lamp before you are ready to cure the gel nail?
    a. Product will soften.   c. Product will harden.
    b. Product will thicken.   d. Product will liquefy.   _____

13. UV gel #3 is referred to as:
    a. base coat gel   c. builder gel
    b. primer coat gel   d. sealer gel   _____

14. UV gels should be rebalanced:
    a. every month   c. when they need it
    b. every week   d. every 2 to 3 weeks _____

15. What is the best way to remove UV gels?
    a. reducing thickness with medium grit abrasive
    b. soaking in acetone to soften product
    c. gently scraping them off using a wooden pusher
    d. all answers   _____

16. Every layer of a UV gel nail enhancement must:
    a. have sealer applied   c. be exposed to UV light
    b. nothing   d. be allowed to air dry _____

17. Oligomers are in between _____ and _____.
    a. a medium, strong hold   c. monomers, polymers
       product
    b. a liquid, a gel   d. a liquid, a solid   _____

18. UV gel #2 is referred to as:
    a. builder UV gel   c. inhibition layer
    b. base coat UV gel   d. finisher UV gel   _____

19. When handling the tacky layer of the UV gel, what precaution(s) apply?
    a. Avoid skin contact.   c. No precautions are
                                     needed.
    b. Nail should be scrubbed.   d. All tacky material must be
                                     removed.   _____

20. _____ are made from either urethane acrylate or urethane methacrylate.
   a. Oligomers   c. Polymers
   b. Monomers   d. Primers   _____

21. Which answer most accurately describes UV gel odor?
   a. very little odor   c. no odor
   b. strong odor   d. depends on the brand   _____

22. For best results, it is important to:
   a. use the strongest bulb you can find
   b. cure the nails for additional time
   c. change your bulbs every other week
   d. use the lamp designed for your UV gel nail system   _____

23. UV bulbs need to be changed when:
   a. they are no longer blue   c. your clients' nails are not curing properly
   b. they flicker   d. you follow a regular replacement schedule   _____

24. What are you risking when you undercure UV gel nails?
   a. service breakdown   c. client defection
   b. skin irritation   d. all answers   _____

25. UV gels are _____ acrylics.
   a. harder than   c. the same as
   b. softer than   d. cannot compare the two   _____

CHAPTER 19—THE CREATIVE TOUCH

1. Why should you get involved in nail art?
   a. It is creative.
   b. It sets your work apart.
   c. It is an effective marketing tool.
   d. All answers.   _____

2. Being open-minded, exposing yourself to all avenues of art services, always listening to your clients, and _____ are the guiding rules of nail art.
   a. there are no such things as mistakes
   b. find a design you like and stick to it
   c. play it safe with your designs
   d. always push the envelope   _____

3. Competitively pricing your nail art begins with:
   a. doing additional art steps at no charge
   b. learning what other technicians are charging
   c. using more than one color
   d. charging $5 less   _____

4. Polished nails should always be _____ before applying artwork.
   a. slightly wet
   b. recleaned
   c. completely dry
   d. opaque   _____

5. The circular color guides that show primary, secondary, tertiary, and complementary colors are called:
   a. color combinations
   b. color gradations
   c. color wheels
   d. color palettes   _____

6. The four color classifications of the color wheel are: primary, secondary, tertiary, and:
   a. analogous
   b. complementary
   c. complimentary
   d. pastel combinations   _____

7. Define complementary colors.
   a. a color scheme incorporating opposite hues on the color wheel
   b. a color scheme incorporating similar hues on the color wheel
   c. a color palette involving colors that make each other look great
   d. a color palette of clashing colors   _____

8. The midsection of the bristles is called the:
   a. thorax
   b. sternum
   c. abdomen
   d. belly   _____

9. The metal band surrounding the brush is called a:
   a. bracelet   c. brace
   b. ferrule   d. brush belly   _____

10. Use the end of a wooden pusher dipped in _____ to apply small gemstones to the nail.
    a. nail art glue   c. nail art polish
    b. base coat   d. nail art sealer   _____

11. When doing a foiling technique, you begin by applying:
    a. ordinary household glue   c. a thin coat of foil adhesive
    b. base coat   d. nail wrap adhesive   _____

12. Another name for a gold leafing sheet is a:
    a. nugget sheet   c. nugget foil
    b. leafd.   tissue foil   _____

13. A basic set of brushes is made up of liner, striper, round, fan, and _____ brushes.
    a. detailer and pointer   c. square and flat
    b. flat and detailer   d. detailer and nondetailer   _____

14. When you pull the brush across the paint surface, what do you create?
    a. fluid strokes   c. crisp line
    b. wider stripe   d. uneven results   _____

15. When using an airbrush device, compressed air is drawn from:
    a. an oxygen container   c. carbon dioxide
    b. the room   d. outside the salon   _____

16. The airbrush system system designed for _____ usually has a well or small color cup.
    a. bottom feed paint   c. gravity-fed paint
    b. dual turbo paint   d. battery operated paint   _____

17. When you are airbrushing properly, the stream of paint is:
    a. highly visible   c. invisible
    b. rich in color   d. noticeably thick   _____

18. Once you are able to _____, you are ready to practice airbrushing on plastic nails.
    a. paint with no overspray   c. draw a straight grid
    b. place a dot in the center   d. create thick and thin lines
       of a square   _____

19. When airbrushing, you should:
    a. brace the gun with your wrist and forearm
    b. move your arm, but keep your wrist straight
    c. bend your wrist, keep your arm straight
    d. move only your wrist   _____

20. When applying paint on the nails correctly, the paint should appear:
    a. dull and powdery   c. shiny and lustrous
    b. slightly iridescent   d. wet looking   _____

21. What is double loading?
    a. placing two colors in a   c. marbleizing
       reservoir
    b. two colors, one on either   d. double dipping
       side of the brush   _____

22. The top secret for selling nail art is:
    a. encouraging clients to be more creative
    b. giving away nail art for the first three months
    c. never practicing on clients
    d. introducing the right design to the right client   _____

23. The end of the brush bristle is called the:
    a. point   c. ferrule
    b. tip   d. belly   _____

24. How do you create a tertiary color?
    a. Mix equal parts of two primary colors and its nearest
       secondary color.
    b. Mix equal parts of one primary color and one of its nearest
       secondary colors.
    c. Mix equal parts of two primary colors and the farthest
       secondary color.
    d. Mix any three colors.   _____

25. You can create a secondary color by:
    a. mixing equal parts of two tertiary colors
    b. mixing pure pigments together
    c. mixing equal parts of two primary colors together
    d. mixing colors next to each other on the color wheel   _____

26. What are primary colors?
    a. Primary colors are colors located directly opposite each other on the color wheel.
    b. Primary colors are pure pigments that cannot be obtained from mixing any other colors together.
    c. Primary colors result from mixing equal parts of secondary colors.
    d. Primary colors are pure pigments that are obtained only by mixing other colors together. _____

27. Define color theory.
    a. a science that categorizes colors
    b. a working knowledge of colors and how they relate, blend, and complement each other
    c. describes the effects of light and dark and all colors in the universe
    d. artistic interpretation of colors and how they relate to each other _____

28. An air compressor does not contain a:
    a. compressor   c. reservoir
    b. gun   d. brush   _____

29. The most common air pressure used to create nail art is:
    a. 25 to 35 pounds psi (per square inch)
    b. 25 to 35 mph (miles per hour)
    c. 25 to 35 RPMs (revolutions per minute)
    d. 100 cubic feet   _____

30. You should hold the nozzle _____ from the nail.
    a. 3 to 4 inches   c. 1 inch
    b. 6 inches   d. 2 to 3 inches   _____

31. An airbrush system works by:
    a. combining air and paint to form an atomized spray
    b. using straight air that has been compressed very tightly
    c. combining oxygen and water to form an atomized spray
    d. combining air from the room and carbon dioxide that we exhale _____

32. Before applying _____, allow the artwork to dry completely.
    a. top coat   c. ridge filler
    b. nail art sealer   d. primer   _____

33. Floating the bead means:
    a. dropping a generous bead of sealer on the nail plate and floating it across the nail with a brush
    b. forming a very lightweight bead
    c. making the bead perfectly round
    d. using a beaded brush to apply top coat
    _____

34. No matter how outstanding your work may be, it must fit your clients' _____ and _____.
    a. lifestyle, please their significant other
    b. lifestyle, sense of fashion
    c. lifestyle, comfort zone
    d. mind-set, mood
    _____

35. Besides _____, doing nail art can be fun and exciting.
    a. preventing your income from declining
    b. dramatically improving your income
    c. maintaining a steady income
    d. enhancing your income
    _____

CHAPTER 20—SEEKING EMPLOYMENT

1. One of the most important parts of your portfolio is your:
   a. introduction
   b. credit history
   c. employment history
   d. skills inventory   _____

2. When securing employment, one of your most vital tools is your:
   a. personal background
   b. employment portfolio
   c. employment history
   d. personal history   _____

3. Before you can determine where you want to work in the beauty industry, what should you do?
   a. Send out résumés.
   b. Get a manicure at all targeted salons.
   c. Define career goals.
   d. Attend classes.   _____

4. When looking for the right salon, what type of clientele should you be seeking?
   a. those with lots of money
   b. one you are comfortable with
   c. conservative and rigid
   d. trendy and avant-garde   _____

5. What is one of the first things you should do when beginning your job search?
   a. Call a few salons.
   b. Obtain a list of area salons.
   c. Talk to fellow students.
   d. Call for a nail appointment.   _____

6. When observing the salon, you should notice whether nail technicians are:
   a. professional and well groomed
   b. color-coordinated
   c. maintaining their nail stations
   d. wearing uniforms   _____

7. If you are seeking immediate employment, when should you start your job search?
   a. When a salon has an ad in the paper.
   b. When you are licensed.
   c. While you are still a student.
   d. When it is the busy season.   _____

8. One way to determine the type of market a salon is servicing is to:
   a. watch local television
   b. drive by the salon regularly
   c. study trade journals
   d. watch the salon's advertising   _____

9. What are potential employers most concerned with?
   a. your life insurance policy
   b. getting his/her nails done
   c. building a clientele and selling retail
   d. keeping records and doing your family's nails

   _____

10. When you wait until the last minute to look for your first job, what are you most likely to do?
    a. take the first offer
    b. never go to state board
    c. change careers
    d. get the best position available

    _____

11. Your résumé should be how long?
    a. one-half page
    b. one to two pages
    c. no less than three pages
    d. as long as necessary

    _____

12. What should be the primary focus of your résumé?
    a. secondary education
    b. work-related experience
    c. employment record
    d. achievements and accomplishments

    _____

13. When you are preparing for a job interview, what should you be concerned with?
    a. your wardrobe and overall appearance
    b. what the interviewer is wearing
    c. best time of day
    d. whether or not to smoke

    _____

14. Which of the following questions are illegal to ask during an interview?
    a. religion
    b. race
    c. national origin
    d. all answers

    _____

15. What is the maximum length of time you should take to answer an interviewer's question?
    a. 1 minute
    b. all the time you need to explain yourself fully
    c. 3 minutes
    d. 2 minutes

    _____

16. In a multiple-choice test, when two choices are worded differently but say the same thing, they both must be:
    a. correct
    b. incorrect
    c. acceptable
    d. logical

    _____

17. What is the stem of a question?
    a. basic question
    b. challenge
    c. answer
    d. nothing important

    _____

18. What is the best way to prepare for an exam?
    a. cramming the morning of the test
    b. avoiding studying two days before
    c. playing mood music while studying
    d. avoiding cramming the night before _____

19. Preparing for a test by practicing good time management skills and having good study habits is called:
    a. being organized   c. being obsessive
    b. being test-wise   d. being test-anxious _____

20. After interviewing, how should you contact the interviewer and/or owner?
    a. Write a thank-you note.   c. Send him/her your picture.
    b. Drop him/her an email to   d. Talk to the receptionist to
       say "Hi."   find out how you did. _____

CHAPTER 21—ON THE JOB

1. The first thing to remember when you are in a service business is that your business revolves around:
   a. making your manager happy
   b. making friends
   c. serving your clients
   d. making a lot of money ____

2. Which entry-level job is appropriate for a newly licensed employee?
   a. manager
   b. employee trainer
   c. entry-level nail technician
   d. nail director ____

3. You should always put your clients:
   a. last
   b. on your list of important things
   c. near the top of your priorities
   d. first ____

4. You are acting respectfully toward your clients and _____ by being punctual and arriving ready to begin work.
   a. neighbors
   b. husband
   c. coworkers
   d. children ____

5. Which of the following pertains to your job description?
   a. duties and responsibilities
   b. calendar of activities
   c. schedule of time off
   d. personal budget ____

6. When taking your first job, the best type of compensation is:
   a. tips plus salary
   b. salary plus commission
   c. cash
   d. straight commission ____

7. Tips are:
   a. taxable up to $400
   b. declared but not taxed
   c. reported as income
   d. not declared or taxed ____

8. The best way to keep tabs on your progress is to ask for feedback. This is called:
   a. a job referral
   b. a client feedback form
   c. an employee evaluation
   d. a coworker comment sheet ____

9. Developing excellent work habits and skills by choosing a role model:
   a. may be limiting
   b. may be competitive
   c. diminishes who are you
   d. is helpful to becoming excellent in your own right ____

10. Striving to help, pitch in, share knowledge, and remain positive
    are all signs of a:
    a. team player   c. problem solver
    b. complainer   d. good client   _____

11. The best way to estimate income and keep track of expenses
    is by having:
    a. a mortgage   c. a budget
    b. a tax return   d. a retirement plan   _____

12. Raising your prices on an annual basis does what?
    a. loses clients   c. loses money
    b. helps to keep pace with d. lets you know you have
       inflation   arrived   _____

13. You are _____ when you do not pay back a loan as
    promised.
    a. in default   c. depressed
    b. in good standing   d. efficient   _____

14. Once a client has decided to purchase a product, stop:
    a. mentioning benefits c. smiling
    b. talking   d. pointing   _____

15. When you have your client book his or her next appointment
    before leaving the salon, you are:
    a. rebooking   c. marketing
    b. prebooking   d. referring   _____

16. You are _____ when you recommend the right retail
    products.
    a. hard selling   c. thinking about your retail
                               commission
    b. soft selling   d. practicing good client care   _____

17. Your _____ consists of clients that see you on a regular
    basis.
    a. core clients   c. fundamental clients
    b. clientele   d. followers   _____

18. You can only become a proficient salesperson when you act:
    a. eager   c. aggressive
    b. confident   d. assertive   _____

19. Define upselling or ticket upgrading.
    a. recommending and selling additional services to your clients
    b. increasing the number of services
    c. selling for the future
    d. not letting a client leave without buying a product
    ____

20. In a salon situation, you must put the needs of the _____ and _____ first.
    a. salon, clients
    b. salon, coworkers
    c. salon, receptionist
    d. manager, salon
    ____

21. In the salon, scheduling is _____ to the day-to-day operations of the business.
    a. central
    b. everything
    c. peripheral
    d. not so important
    ____

22. Even the most ideal job will have its:
    a. heartbreak
    b. pain
    c. benefits
    d. challenges
    ____

23. You can perfect your _____ while working in a salon.
    a. life skills
    b. customer care skills
    c. salon skills
    d. self skills
    ____

24. Team members realize that you cannot fulfill your work potential:
    a. with a group
    b. alone
    c. without a manager
    d. without walk-ins
    ____

25. You must have _____ in order to perform your duties and do what is expected of you.
    a. a list of recommended classes
    b. a copy of your appointments
    c. good communication
    d. a written job description
    ____

CHAPTER 22—THE SALON BUSINESS

1. The best form of advertising is:
    a. Yellow Pages
    b. Internet
    c. word of mouth
    d. television
    _____

2. The receptionist is called the quarterback of the salon because:
    a. a receptionist physically directs the flow of the salon
    b. a receptionist intercepts problems
    c. a receptionist makes a game plan for the day
    d. all answers
    _____

3. What is word-of-mouth advertising?
    a. free advertisement
    b. personal recommendation
    c. a way to build a clientele by pleasing one client after another
    d. all answers
    _____

4. Each of the following describes entrepreneurial situations except:
    a. booth rental
    b. partnership
    c. sole proprietor
    d. head nail technician
    _____

5. As a booth renter, you are responsible for all of the following except:
    a. paying for all education
    b. managing and paying for inventory
    c. paying all taxes, including higher Social Security
    d. maintaining the salon
    _____

6. Two important elements that create a successful salon are:
    a. having good visibility and accessibility
    b. having all your supplies paid for and your first month's rent covered
    c. having cheap rent and no set store hours
    d. offering quick turnaround on services and promising to do a great job
    _____

7. What is a business plan?
    a. written description of your business as you see it today and as you foresee it in the next 5 years (detailed by year)
    b. written description of your hopes and dreams for your business and where you want to be in 5 years
    c. written description of your business as you see it today and as you believe it will be in the next 5 years
    d. a plan of success that begins with writing down short-term and long-term goals, followed by a goal-setting exercise and a time management program to make them come true _____

8. Identify which of the following is not a business model:
   a. corporation
   b. partnership
   c. sole proprietorship
   d. mayoral department _____

9. A corporation helps protect:
   a. a person's reputation
   b. personal assets
   c. a person's future career
   d. all business assets _____

10. In the event you incur unmanageable debts, a corporation will:
    a. limit monthly payments
    b. limit personal financial liability
    c. protect you from your creditors
    d. prevent you from running into financial trouble _____

11. When purchasing an existing salon, you must have a written agreement that includes:
    a. complete and signed statement of inventory, including the value of each article
    b. written purchase and sale agreement
    c. written agreement of responsibility of existing debt
    d. all answers _____

12. Most salon owners do not own:
    a. the building
    b. their business name
    c. their inventory
    d. their fixtures _____

13. In your lease, you must specify:
    a. who owns the property (stations, etc.) that is physically attached to your space.
    b. whether or not you are able to sublease your space to an independent contractor or new owner
    c. who is responsible for necessary renovations and regular maintenance of the building and grounds
    d. all answers _____

14. When purchasing a salon, what information should be included about the existing clientele?
    a. client contact list
    b. service and visitation records
    c. chemical formulas
    d. all answers _____

15. When you first become a salon owner, it is wise to have a _____ who can give you advice along the way.
    a. circle of contacts
    b. circle of friends
    c. group of paid consultants
    d. circle of salon owners _____

16. A smooth business operation has:
    a. excellent customer service delivery and proper pricing of services
    b. sufficient investment capital and efficiency of management
    c. trained salon personnel and good business procedures
    d. all answers ____

17. Your bookkeeping system must keep track of:
    a. service sales   c. income and expenses
    b. retail sales   d. employee attendance ____

18. Client service records should include:
    a. dates of visits, services received, formulas, retail purchases, client feedback, and any special products used for the services
    b. dates of visits and services received
    c. dates of visits, services, retail purchases, and whether or not they were prebooked
    d. formulas ____

19. To own a successful salon, your business must:
    a. be sparkling clean, be physically attractive, and run smoothly
    b. be the most popular in the area
    c. be the most progressive
    d. have the best receptionist ____

20. Layout is crucial to having:
    a. a profitable salon   c. a happy clientele
    b. a physically smooth   d. an injury-free situation
       running operation ____

Part II: Answers to Exam Review for Nail Technology

CHAPTER 1—HISTORY AND OPPORTUNITIES

1. a	6. d	11. a	16. d
2. b	7. d	12. b	17. d
3. d	8. a	13. a	
4. c	9. d	14. a	
5. d	10. a	15. b	

CHAPTER 2—LIFE SKILLS

1. d	7. a	13. c	19. b	25. b
2. a	8. b	14. d	20. b	26. b
3. a	9. d	15. a	21. d	27. b
4. d	10. d	16. a	22. c	28. d
5. b	11. d	17. b	23. a	29. b
6. d	12. d	18. a	24. c	30. c

CHAPTER 3—YOUR PROFESSIONAL IMAGE

1. c	7. a	13. b	19. a	25. d
2. a	8. b	14. c	20. a	26. c
3. d	9. d	15. d	21. a	27. b
4. c	10. a	16. d	22. d	
5. d	11. c	17. b	23. c	
6. d	12. a	18. c	24. c	

CHAPTER 4—COMMUNICATING FOR SUCCESS

1. b	6. a	11. c	16. a	21. b
2. b	7. c	12. a	17. c	22. b
3. d	8. b	13. d	18. b	23. b
4. d	9. d	14. b	19. d	24. a
5. b	10. a	15. c	20. c	25. d

CHAPTER 5—INFECTION CONTROL: PRINCIPLES AND PRACTICES

1. a	8. d	15. a	22. a	29. a
2. b	9. b	16. a	23. a	30. d
3. c	10. d	17. c	24. b	31. a
4. a	11. c	18. a	25. b	32. d
5. b	12. c	19. b	26. a	33. a
6. c	13. b	20. b	27. d	34. d
7. a	14. b	21. c	28. b	35. c

CHAPTER 6—GENERAL ANATOMY AND PHYSIOLOGY

1. c	13. a	25. d	37. c	49. a
2. d	14. a	26. c	38. d	50. a
3. b	15. c	27. b	39. c	51. c
4. c	16. a	28. b	40. a	52. a
5. b	17. a	29. d	41. b	53. c
6. a	18. c	30. b	42. d	54. d
7. a	19. b	31. a	43. b	55. b
8. a	20. a	32. d	44. d	56. a
9. c	21. b	33. d	45. b	57. b
10. d	22. c	34. b	46. c	58. b
11. b	23. a	35. d	47. c	59. b
12. b	24. a	36. b	48. b	60. b

CHAPTER 7—SKIN STRUCTURE AND GROWTH

1. d	11. b	21. c	31. a	41. c
2. a	12. d	22. b	32. c	42. d
3. a	13. a	23. b	33. d	43. d
4. a	14. b	24. c	34. c	44. c
5. d	15. c	25. d	35. b	
6. c	16. a	26. c	36. b	
7. d	17. d	27. b	37. d	
8. a	18. d	28. d	38. d	
9. b	19. c	29. b	39. a	
10. b	20. a	30. d	40. b	

CHAPTER 8—NAIL STRUCTURE AND GROWTH

1. b	6. b	11. b	16. a	21. a
2. b	7. c	12. d	17. d	22. d
3. d	8. d	13. c	18. a	23. b
4. b	9. d	14. a	19. c	24. a
5. d	10. b	15. a	20. d	

CHAPTER 9—NAIL DISEASES AND DISORDERS

1. b	9. a	17. d	25. d	33. b
2. d	10. d	18. d	26. b	34. a
3. a	11. b	19. c	27. c	35. d
4. c	12. d	20. d	28. d	36. d
5. b	13. c	21. c	29. c	37. c
6. a	14. a	22. b	30. b	
7. d	15. b	23. a	31. b	
8. c	16. c	24. b	32. d	

CHAPTER 10—BASICS OF CHEMISTRY

1. b	8. d	15. a	22. d	29. c
2. b	9. a	16. b	23. b	30. d
3. a	10. b	17. a	24. c	31. c
4. b	11. a	18. d	25. a	32. b
5. d	12. d	19. b	26. d	33. d
6. b	13. d	20. d	27. b	34. a
7. b	14. b	21. a	28. b	35. b

CHAPTER 11—NAIL PRODUCT CHEMISTRY SIMPLIFIED

1. b	13. d	25. a	37. d	49. d
2. a	14. d	26. a	38. c	50. c
3. d	15. d	27. d	39. b	51. b
4. b	16. b	28. b	40. a	52. d
5. a	17. d	29. a	41. c	53. b
6. c	18. c	30. a	42. b	54. b
7. a	19. a	31. b	43. b	55. d
8. a	20. c	32. b	44. d	56. a
9. d	21. c	33. b	45. a	
10. a	22. d	34. c	46. b	
11. b	23. a	35. a	47. a	
12. b	24. b	36. d	48. b	

CHAPTER 12—BASICS OF ELECTRICITY

1. c	9. d	17. b	25. c	33. a
2. b	10. a	18. a	26. a	34. b
3. a	11. d	19. b	27. b	35. b
4. b	12. a	20. c	28. d	36. d
5. d	13. b	21. c	29. b	37. b
6. b	14. c	22. d	30. d	38. a
7. c	15. b	23. d	31. c	
8. d	16. b	24. a	32. a	

CHAPTER 13—MANICURING

1. d	9. d	17. c	25. c	33. b
2. a	10. d	18. c	26. b	34. d
3. b	11. b	19. c	27. d	35. c
4. d	12. b	20. d	28. d	36. a
5. a	13. d	21. b	29. d	37. c
6. d	14. b	22. b	30. c	38. a
7. a	15. b	23. d	31. d	39. c
8. a	16. b	24. c	32. c	

CHAPTER 14—PEDICURING

1. d	6. b	11. c	16. b	21. b
2. b	7. a	12. b	17. b	22. a
3. a	8. b	13. a	18. c	23. a
4. d	9. a	14. d	19. c	24. c
5. d	10. a	15. c	20. a	25. a

CHAPTER 15—ELECTRIC FILING

1. c	9. a	17. c	25. a	33. b
2. a	10. c	18. c	26. b	34. b
3. d	11. b	19. a	27. b	35. c
4. b	12. c	20. d	28. a	36. d
5. a	13. a	21. b	29. a	
6. b	14. c	22. d	30. b	
7. a	15. d	23. c	31. a	
8. b	16. d	24. d	32. c	

CHAPTER 16—NAIL TIPS, WRAPS, AND NO-LIGHT GELS

1. b	8. b	15. a	22. b	29. b
2. d	9. c	16. d	23. b	30. a
3. b	10. a	17. b	24. b	31. a
4. d	11. c	18. c	25. a	32. c
5. d	12. a	19. a	26. a	33. b
6. b	13. c	20. d	27. d	34. d
7. c	14. b	21. c	28. c	35. d

CHAPTER 17—ACRYLIC (METHACRYLATE) NAIL ENHANCEMENTS

1. a	9. b	17. a	25. a	33. a
2. b	10. a	18. b	26. b	34. a
3. b	11. c	19. a	27. d	35. d
4. a	12. c	20. b	28. b	36. b
5. d	13. d	21. b	29. c	37. d
6. c	14. a	22. d	30. c	
7. b	15. d	23. b	31. c	
8. a	16. d	24. a	32. a	

CHAPTER 18—UV GELS

1. d	6. a	11. b	16. c	21. a
2. b	7. b	12. c	17. d	22. d
3. d	8. c	13. d	18. a	23. d
4. b	9. a	14. d	19. a	24. d
5. d	10. d	15. d	20. a	25. b

CHAPTER 19—THE CREATIVE TOUCH

1. d	8. d	15. b	22. d	29. a
2. a	9. b	16. c	23. b	30. d
3. b	10. d	17. c	24. b	31. a
4. c	11. c	18. b	25. c	32. b
5. c	12. a	19. b	26. b	33. a
6. b	13. b	20. a	27. b	34. c
7. a	14. a	21. b	28. d	35. d

CHAPTER 20—SEEKING EMPLOYMENT

1. d	6. a	11. b	16. b
2. b	7. c	12. d	17. a
3. c	8. d	13. a	18. d
4. b	9. c	14. d	19. b
5. b	10. a	15. d	20. a

CHAPTER 21—ON THE JOB

1. c	6. a	11. c	16. d	21. a
2. c	7. c	12. b	17. b	22. d
3. d	8. c	13. a	18. b	23. b
4. c	9. d	14. b	19. a	24. b
5. a	10. a	15. a	20. a	25. d

CHAPTER 22—THE SALON BUSINESS

1. c	6. a	11. d	16. d
2. d	7. a	12. a	17. c
3. d	8. d	13. d	18. a
4. d	9. b	14. d	19. a
5. d	10. b	15. a	20. b

NOTES

NOTES

NOTES

NOTES

NOTES